FLIPPED

A DRUG-INDUCED JOURNEY TO THE
EVENT HORIZON OF INSANITY

FLIPPED

A Drug-induced Journey to The Event Horizon of Insanity

Robert P. Cantu

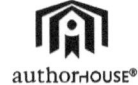

AuthorHouse™
1663 Liberty Drive
Bloomington, IN 47403
www.authorhouse.com
Phone: 1-800-839-8640

First published by AuthorHouse   08/12/2011

ISBN: 978-1-4634-4830-1 (sc)
ISBN: 978-1-4634-4829-5 (hc)
ISBN: 978-1-4634-4828-8 (ebk)

Library of Congress Control Number: 2011914179

Printed in the United States of America

Contents

Acknowledgements

As one can expect, no book is ever completed in a vacuum or completely by one person. This book was written as a consequence of an unexpected turn of events from a moderate illness to hospitalization and descent into a black hole of mental deterioration. I would like to thank Diana, and especially those Charlotte doctors who treated me effectively and offered additional information relative to my illness and mental health. Any errors with medical information, book content, or chronology are strictly of my doing, and I bear full responsibility.

Dedication

This book is dedicated to Diana Fowler and Dolores S. Cantu, my mother, for the love, wisdom, and strength they demonstrated during my short-term psychosis. Diana, especially, who inspired me to better mental and physical health by suggesting and recommending many things that quickly put me on the path to recovery. To my sister, Dr. Margaret Cantu, my brother, Jesse M. Cantu, and several local doctors (a cardiologist, gastroenterologist, internist, neurologist, psychologist, and psychiatrist), I give my thanks for their individual support and understanding.

"Do not go gentle into that good night."
—Dylan Thomas

Introduction

Today in astrophysics, there is a theory that once you enter the event horizon of a black hole escape is impossible because of intense gravity. This is a true story of how I entered the event horizon of a mental black hole, but through a medical systems approach to treatment, I avoided being committed. Today, every once in a while when I exceed my physical or mental limitations, I flirt with that past mental state.

How we are medically treated successfully, or not, along the perilous trail of mental health determines whether we are institutionalized. It seemed inevitable I would end up in a loony bin; however, only one of the nine doctors I met along the way of my treatment alluded to that. You'd think my confidence would soar after knowing that only one out of nine doctors thought me potentially certifiable; not so. The rest believed I would end up being quite sane, but that remained to be determined.

If you have experienced severe acute anxiety, mild catatonia, panic disorders, paranoia, agoraphobia, or any other form of mental illness, this book is for you. So, step right up, and let me share my condition, which none of us should ever have to experience.

Robert P. Cantu
2011

Chapter 1

How It All Started

It was right after the weekend of the 2005 New Year holiday, a Jane Eyre-type winter day. At lunch, I had eaten soup with a lot of okra with those large, slimy seeds, and later that night, I ate a fruit tart containing a cornucopia of fruits and nuts and had probably not taken in sufficient quantities of water or tea. That's when the whole miserable event began. At work the next morning, I felt feverish, and while speaking on the phone, low voices and sounds began increasing in volume. This was turning out to be one of my very worst days. I couldn't decide whether to go to see my doctor that day or wait it out.

Procrastinating has always been a virtue and science for me; sometimes I can be so indecisive. It was just a slight fever, anyway, and I had no pain. I wondered if the flu shot from the previous week had not taken, and I was coming down with the flu. Who would have known what lay in store for me then and for the rest of that year?

A late afternoon conference call with several of my Canadian colleagues forced me to decide that I would stay through the dreary afternoon instead of visiting my doctor. I went home at the usual time with that slight fever, and around 7:00 p.m., a dull pain started on my left, lower side. Later in the evening, the pain intensified, as well as my fever, which now hovered around one hundred degrees Fahrenheit. The pain started to course throughout my body. My normal body temperature being 97.6 degrees Fahrenheit, over one hundred degrees was not terribly high for me, but it was still a concern. Because I'd had a similar occurrence five years earlier diagnosed as diverticulitis, I knew it to be the same thing.

Realizing it was getting dark and might be too late to reach my internist, I called for him anyway, but I got the evening shift nurse. The best she could do after reviewing my records and confirming the probable condition was to recommend that I go to emergency for treatment. The pain and fever could not wait until the next day, when I could go see my doctor. My wife, a very slim, blue-eyed brunette, drove me to the hospital emergency care section.

Still the week of the New Year, I thought the emergency room might be very busy; I toughed it and went in. As I looked over the expanse of the emergency room, it overflowed, wall-to-wall, replete with racial diversity; many faces contorted in pain. Others grimaced with discomfort either from disease, a drug reaction, or overdose. It was a sea of sickness everywhere. What else should I have expected? Even the triage section was overloaded with patients. The check-in staff said that it might be several hours before a doctor could see me. Did I have a choice at this time? No, I was too sick and getting worse by the hour.

I worried that a man sitting next to me with a hacking cough might be a person with a terminal case of tuberculosis. He kept spitting blood and wiping it into an apparently never-cleaned handkerchief. Right then, I stood up and moved away. Just in case, I didn't want to contract another disease and add to my situation and complicate matters; the flu season was at its height. In the next room, a pregnant woman kept her arms around her distended belly in hopes of soothing her premature contractions. She, too, was in pain. And the list continued. Dante's *Inferno* may not have had such a Goya-istic entanglement of writhing bodies in so many stages of pain. Do you blame me for not wanting to sit next to the cough? Christ, even the large sofas in an adjoining room bulged over with sick people accompanied by their relatives, so I stood against the wall for a long time. Finally, at 1:00 a.m., a nurse called me up, took my vitals, had me change into a gown, and moved me to a small, temporary room. That's when the check-in and preliminaries began.

The very small room had the basic vitals-monitoring equipment, yet it was crammed with only a gurney on which to lie down. This was to be my interim room, as no hospital room was available at the time. In other words, I'd need to stay in the room to be examined and medicated. By 4:00 a.m., the pain and fever had increased so that I was extremely uncomfortable, while the hard, metal gurney added to my increasing discomfort. My back was now hurting so I couldn't find a tolerable position. In the meantime, my blood was taken for routine blood chemistries.

Later, technicians took several chest X-rays and a magnetic resonance imaging (MRI) scan to view the colon. I had to take the fluorescent orange-colored viscous liquid for the contrast agent, and a hell of a lot of it. I think about half a gallon made me nauseous, yet I drank the disgusting stuff; a chilled dye, I'm sure, as if being chilled would mask the bitter, downright disgusting taste.

By around 7:00 that morning, the attending emergency doctor confirmed a high white blood count and diverticulitis, a right inguinal hernia, and other superfluous conditions. A male nurse, close to my height but about twenty pounds heavier, started to add morphine to the IV for my pain and discomfort. Quickly, I asked him the dosage. He related four milligrams, and I immediately asked him to lower it to two milligrams, as I had an overactive immune system and had no desire to be comatose. He granted my request. It should be noted that I had pain, but certainly not enough to double me over yet or warrant such a high dose of morphine.

Another nurse, quite petite and young, came in shortly, and she administered, through the existing IV line, both Tequin (fluoroquinolone) and Flagyl (metronidazole), which were ordered by the emergency care doctor. Because Tequin was new to me, I asked the nurse what it was. Past allergic reactions to antibiotics and other significant medications had always caused me concern with new drugs.

She said, "It's one of our better antibiotics prescribed to patients who have abdominal infections." I nodded to her and felt a little sleepy by then, but I had trouble sleeping. Who could really sleep with all the activity, vitals being constantly taken, and interruptions out the yin yang?

Up until this time, I had considered myself well versed in pharmacology, having majored in zoology and chemistry in college, and while in the navy, I took several pharmaceutical courses through Johns Hopkins Medical School and read the *Physician's Desk Reference* like a classical novel, but I had not known what fluoroquinolone was, nor could I spell it, but I did know about Flagyl. In an earlier bout with diverticulitis, Flagyl had been tag-teamed with another antibiotic to eliminate the disease. During 1998, fluoroquinolones were going through the approval rating with the FDA, which is why I was unfamiliar with those kinds of antibiotics.

By late that afternoon, a regular room became available for me. The bed was such a comfort after spending over fifteen hours on a stiff, metal gurney that I fell immediately to sleep, only to be awakened by yet another staff visitor.

At about 5:30 p.m., the hospital administrator came to my room and said, "I want to apologize for taking so long to get you a room, but as you know, this is the busy time of the year. Well, with the New Year and all." Although I thanked him, I was still put out with the whole discomfort thing, having been strapped to the hard gurney way too long, and I wanted to verbally pummel him with multiple cuss words. Maybe I should have waited and gone to see my doctor.

After he left, I could feel myself starting to improve mentally, despite the many interruptions of being administered medicines and their not allowing me to sleep. I thought to myself, *Ah geez, let me rest for crying out loud.* The last time I had had sleep of any consequence was Sunday night. Here it was already three days later, I was sick and physically exhausted, add to this I hadn't eaten anything for over twenty-four hours, and I was now feeling dizzy and weak from hunger. The diet for a diverticulitis patient, I was to find out, consisted of nothing but soup, crackers, and those kinds of things that don't give you any calories so that you feel even more miserable. Maybe I should have paid someone to bring me real food so I could have recovered sooner.

The next morning, the hospital dietician, a very attractive dark-haired woman in her mid-thirties, I guessed, lectured me on what I should eat and drink. Oh, she was cute, you bet. Being slightly delirious, I wished I could have met her earlier in my life and under different circumstances.

The dietician had so much good stuff to tell me—a veritable fountain of information—that I wanted her to stay all day and tell me everything she knew. With my I-know-all-that-crap-already attitude, my eyes glazed over, and I really didn't learn anything new, but she reminded me of things I should be doing for better health. Seriously, though, I was lucid enough and paid attention to her stressing the importance of drinking a minimum of eight glasses of water a day and eating sufficient fiber every day, whatever that meant. Admittedly, those recommendations stayed with me and would prove to be important in my recovery and sustained health.

Later that day, the doctor who had seen me in the emergency room was my attending physician. He confirmed my recurrent diverticulitis. He added that I had an empty space on my right inguinal side. I mentioned that it was most probably a recurrent hernia.

He said, "Try to minimize any straining. That will reduce any further complications with your hernia. It may also help with your diverticulitis. Keep in mind intermittent abdominal straining can lead to complications. Excessive pressure could exacerbate or launch other conditions like hemorrhoids and fissures that could result in abdominal discomfort. I wouldn't want you straining like Elvis did prior to his passing." I wholeheartedly agreed with him and realized that could help in reducing any further flare-ups with my diverticulitis.

Chapter 2

If at First You Don't Succeed

In retrospect, I now appreciate why a slow intravenous fluid dosage dripping through a catheter in my left arm vein would not produce any side effects. In that manner, you don't receive the whole dosage in one shot or pill. An IV is generally a slow titration of a medicine. Through the IV, the antibiotic quickly killed most of the bacteria that caused the infection, and simultaneously, the white count receded in my blood as well. No question, the antibiotic was working.

Knowing that the disease was under control, my doctor released me from the hospital that Thursday morning. I was elated, feeling great, and I could resume doing my usual sixty push-ups every other day and other exercises. Mainly, I would get back to work.

Once released from the hospital on January 6, I began taking a one thousand-milligram Tequin pill twice a day, together with Flagyl. Unfortunately, it took only twenty-four hours for a few adverse events to start manifesting themselves. Per standard pharmacy regimen, common side effects were already acknowledged and published in the toxicology handout for this specific antibiotic, Tequin, but I was so overpowered by the mounting side effects that I had not read the handout carefully, but Diana had and subsequently may have been the reason I'm alive today and able to write this personal narrative. Almost to the published word as she described to me, I experienced all of the side effects and more; however, some of the not so common ones that came on later may have been caused by other medicines prescribed to counter the Tequin's initial deleterious effects.

Either way, it made little difference; I was screwed coming and going. And incredibly, this was only the first week of my illness, and those published side effects started to materialize right before me and disabled me physically and mentally in the coming days, weeks, and months.

With being home for only twenty-four hours, on late Friday night, as I was trying to sleep, what seemed like a powerful jackhammer hit me in the center of the chest. I sprang out of bed frightened out of my wits and immediately assumed that I was in the midst of a heart attack. Another power thump startled me, and I grew enormously anxious. I called to my wife, who was asleep, woke her up, and briefed her; she dressed immediately, and we were back to the emergency room. I now had heart palpitations, a very fast pulse rate, and mounting anxiety over this new condition along with pain, which was still my Coleridge's albatross—diverticulitis. Water fountains and bottled water were everywhere, but I couldn't drink a damn drop. The pain in my lower left abdomen mounted while high anxiety—I was sweating with an overwhelming feeling that I was about to "pack it in"—was making me jump out of my skin while trying to paralyze me. My blood pressure was surely over the top at that moment.

Describing my immediate health state to the attending nurse, I was checked in swiftly without waiting, as I was now considered a heart patient, not unusual for a man my age. Had I experienced a heart attack with maybe another on its way? A laundry list of heart tests were started, including blood enzymes to determine if the heart enzymes were elevated, a positive test confirming a heart attack. My attending emergency doctor, an attractive woman with curly, blonde hair and medium build who wore blue, plastic Crocs, and another assistant doctor reviewed the blood tests with me. My wife was sitting next to me as my advocate. She suspected that I was too confused by this time in my illness to make a lot of sense. Without question, she was right. I was mad, too, now believing I had experienced a heart attack for whatever reasons I wasn't sure, but I had a major suspicion. The possibility that the medicine being prescribed might be at fault entered my mind. I desperately hoped it wasn't my heart or a blood clot traveling through my blood stream.

The attending doctor confirmed that my blood enzymes were normal. A relief, but my blood pressure was still an extremely high

186/100 with a pulse rate of over 100. My ECG was normal, so no apparent heart attack had occurred. But what was causing these adverse side effects?

I thought this all through while the doctors were conferring. What I concluded and then articulated to them came out as if I were viewing everyone from the ceiling. I said, "This chest condition started with taking Tequin in pill form. My blood pressure and pulse have always been on the low side, and my wife will confirm that." She looked over to the doctor and nodded in agreement.

I went on. "In fact a month ago, after being on Lipitor for six months, a blood test confirmed that my liver enzymes were normal. My blood pressure was 120/68 and pulse rate 65. Those are good numbers for someone in his early sixties. I'm not going to take the damn Tequin anymore. It's got to be causing these horrific side effects. I'm not on anything else, except Lipitor!"

The doctor countered without wavering. "You need to stay on Tequin. I'll treat your side effects. We know how to treat them." I didn't know at the time that "there are no known antidotes to quickly reverse a quinolone reaction," according to *Medication Sense*, by Jay S. Cohen, MD. Somehow I had a feeling that the ER doctor was lying or hadn't known what she was saying. I was beginning to believe that she thought I was some inconsequential dilettante when it came to health and medicine. Well, it was true to a certain point. Yet, I knew something she didn't: my body and mind. In all my years of visiting doctors for whatever ailment, I had never felt coerced to take a drug like I had with this ER doctor. Even though the air was heavy with the scent of hexachlorophene, it was going to be a lot heavier with the scent of conflict coming on, and I dug in my heels.

Staring her in the face and thinking, "*Bullshit you'll control the side effects,*" I said, "You didn't hear me. I'm not taking Tequin anymore." I couldn't believe this. I lay there guarded and mystified why she thought she could treat my side effects not even comprehending what they were or how they occurred. Was I really in a hospital, or was I dreaming?

Sitting there and taking this all in, my wife spoke up and said, "Bob's not had much sleep. He's been sick now for over a week and feeling really bad. He may be a little off the radar of conscious perception." In simpler words, they thought I was a little out of it.

I rolled my eyes in obvious disagreement but decided to hold my tongue, for I was still with the program, and then said, "Diana read the Tequin side effects published on the Internet, and she agrees with the Tequin pharmaceutical handout that these new conditions are a direct result of the antibiotic, especially my heart palpitations, very high blood pressure, and unbelievable anxiety."

The article Diana had read the night before came from the Tequin pharmaceutical handout, and it read:

> Since its release, Tequin has become one of the most frequently prescribed antibiotics on the market; however, it has severe side effects and may cause issues with **severe blood sugar changes,** including low-blood sugar (hypoglycemia) and high-blood sugar (hyperglycemia). **Heart side effects** can be changes in the QT sinal waves that can be permanent heart palpitations and possible arterial fibrillation. **Serious allergic reactions**, which may be fatal, include trouble breathing, throat closure, and inflammation of the lips, tongue, or face. **Central nervous system side effects** such as dizziness, tremors, confusion, depression, hallucination, or suicidal thoughts can occur independently or in combination. **Rupture of a tendon** in the ankle or foot may occur which may cause severe pain and inflammation, and **severe diarrhea** can occur which may be fatal.

With an unbending tone and with hard eyes staring at me in an effort to manipulate me, the emergency doctor said, "You need to stay on Tequin or you will lose a part of your colon." No soft tone or compassion, yet in her straightaway, unpolished bedside manner,

I knew she was right about the colon but wrong about the antibiotic. It had to be changed.

Stubbornly holding my ground and keeping my defense shield up, I said, "I'd rather lose a portion of my colon than become disabled or possibly die of complications if I were to stay on Tequin."

To say she was very unhappy with my decision was an understatement, for her body language revealed to me everything I needed to know. Quickly, she left the examination room in a huff. There hovered in the air a silence so heavy that it smothered me and held on for what seemed like an eternity. I never saw her again, nor did I get her name. Her attitude wreaked "her way or the highway." She had no idea what was up with Tequin, nor did any of us know its full negative consequences or how it would play out, at least in my case.

Though many things went through my mind with this doctor, one thing that stood out was the consideration that when you die in the hospital, most likely it was the "will of God." What a bunch of esoteric hogwash! Where is the responsibility that the doctor, a specific medication, or one of the nurses or technicians, of course not intentionally, may have caused the death? No one is infallible, period. What I mean is that, first of all, a drug company together with its biochemists formulated the drug, and a doctor insisted that I continue on the drug irrespective if it could go on to disable me or possibly kill me. Would that have been God who killed me? I don't think so. So just how many patients die in a hospital due to poor drug management, some allergic reaction, or some deficiency in medical practice skills? The answer may never be known. But what is clear is that "Medication side effects is the number four leading cause of death in the U.S. annually", according to the *Journal of the American Medical Association, JAMA 1998 April 15;279(15):1200-5.*

If you'd ask me what my assessment of the ER doctor was, I'd have to say that she didn't have my best interests at heart. How could someone when they didn't really know me, or my medical history of allergic reaction to a number of prescribed drugs? She completely discounted that I had experienced a negative reaction to the antibiotic. Also, was Tequin vetted and tested carefully by the FDA before it was approved in 1999? This was 2005, and Tequin, a synthetic fluoroquinolone antibiotic, had been on the market for only five years with a trail a mile long of medical issues.

Fortunately the emergency doctor, however gruff with me, did have presence of mind to have me admitted to the hospital, because I was still exhibiting an elevated blood pressure, high pulse rate, fever, and pain, and her attending medical team had no idea what was wrong with me. They would not concede that Tequin could be the cause. I found out later that the hospital never reconciled the possibility that Tequin was at fault; talk about no comment.

Because my condition was believed to still be a heart issue and in actuality a diagnostic conundrum, I was assigned to the coronary section of the hospital. If these things didn't cause enough pain and discomfort, the electrodes to monitor my heart condition and rate were set with latex. I'm allergic to latex, and the allergy manifests itself as round, large, red itchy spots. As nurses changed these from day-to-day, circular nodules appeared at every site that looked like leeches had worked me over, or better, a large octopus had had a meal of me. Those sites itched like crazy, but no one changed the application electrode pads to cotton or a nonallergenic fabric. At the time, those circular, red spots about the size of a quarter were not that important in my mind, small potatoes in comparison, but still a concern. A low-salt diet was all I got for a couple of days.

Another doctor was assigned to me the next morning, and she was a tall, slim African American with neatly starched denims. Compared to Miss Congeniality with no bedside manner, this doctor went into detail about my MRI and said, "You do still have the diverticulitis, and I noticed a couple of benign tumors right above your left adrenal gland, which are not a concern at this time."

She further said, "I'm changing you to a sulfa antibiotic. Our records indicate you are allergic to sulfa, so I want you to drink plenty of water with each pill and you should be okay. If you have any adverse effects, stop taking them and call me. By the way, your stress test was negative. We're going to monitor you throughout the day and night. If your blood pressure stabilizes by tomorrow morning, I may release you by the afternoon."

Now what I'm going to say about this new doctor is true, and not because she is an African American and I'm trying to appease the left-wing gods of liberalism. She really *did* have my best interests at heart, and that's my perception of her excellent bedside manner. In fact, I had wished she could have been my emergency doctor going back to January 5, when the first episode began; perhaps the outcome may have been different. Yes, she was sincere and smart. The emergency doctor just wanted to win the argument with me because she thought she knew better. She did know more about medicine; I will admit that, but she didn't know what was better at that time for me. I would be disabled, confined to a mental institution, or dead, and my story would have never been told had I listened to her and remained on Tequin.

Chapter 3

Would Medicines Counter Tequin, or Was I Headed to the Loony Bin?

Pretty much back to normal only from the standpoint of a stable pulse and steady heart rate, I was released that Monday afternoon. I still had close to two weeks of taking the combination of the sulfa antibiotic and Flagyl. However, about two weeks later, I still had diarrhea, was experiencing severe insomnia, had a fever, and my diverticulitis was in full bloom. By then it was early February, and I could not shake my condition and knew the sulfa drug was not working. To complicate matters, it was clear to Diana that I was behaving strangely and beginning to show signs of mental meltdown shortly after the second hospital visit. Even I knew straightaway that I wasn't "right in the head," forgetting for a minute the real illness being the abdominal infection and accompanying physical issues.

What was wrong? I went to see my internist, a family doctor and one whom I had developed a good rapport with. He stood about six feet, was robust, and always took the time to listen. I thought his premature gray hair was a very distinguishing mark for him and gave him that aristocratic and knowledgeable look. I had already been seeing him for a little over ten years. He saw me, heard my issues concerning my anxiety and insomnia, and prescribed Ambien for insomnia; he also put me on Lexapro, a selective serotonin reuptake inhibitor which treats depression and anxiety. Trying to get to the bottom of my mental condition, something he never saw in me until the Tequin episode, he suggested that I might already have had a predisposition to high anxiety but perhaps not depression and panic disorder. I'm not saying he was wrong, but rather on the right track. He felt that I had developed a general anxiety disorder, referred in short as GAD, and expected the Lexapro would put me back to a normal state. I told him how much I thought my mind, at that time, was like a house made of cards; remove one card, and the house would come tumbling down. Alter one chemical or neurotransmitter in my brain, and I too could crumble after only one card removed. And I had. I wondered many times if, although my panic attacks and depression were most probably a biochemical imbalance, the anxieties were more likely a product of my scatterbrain imagination. Was this anxiety based on fear or originated from it? Where did this out-of-control and overblown fear come from? It seemed like I was moments away from going mad, a fact not conjecture.

Could this have been a holdover from a childhood-suppressed event, or the fear of the unknown when our family split up when I was only a year old? I remembered clearly living in Los Angeles and sleeping in my crib or a small bed, and while in the midst of drifting off to sleep, I immediately woke up from something frightful like a loud sound that was never located, but imagined. Was that the sound of a piece of chalk screeching across a blackboard really in my mind? Did this imaginational trauma become a part of me to wind its way throughout my life? The question remains to be answered, if ever.

Consider that for years, my brother and sister and I lived with no father and only a bright, energetic mother who worked herself practically to the bone with over fifty hours a week for a meager wage, working on her only day off to do the laundry, wash dishes, run errands via bus, our only means of transportation then. Yet, with all of that, she was able to attend to us when we needed her. That's all we had then. Did we help? Of course, but what could three young ones do at such tender ages? We did mop and wash the dishes, but because there was never much food in the house, we couldn't cook, nor did we know how, and we had to rely on relatives; however, they were busy with their family ties and lives. I tired of Karo syrup on stale pieces of bread. But then, didn't well-to-dos get tired of steak served too often? Anyway, sometimes bread and Karo syrup is all that we had to eat.

No doubt about it, I was given to horrible, returning nightmares, insecurity, and self-doubt from my very early years. I was one year old, when my mother and father divorced, and the youngest and most vulnerable; so there you have it. Unfortunately, I was a potential nutcase in the making and in the early stages of development. Was there any salvation for me? Was my life fated to insecurity and on the cusp of insanity? I think it was a little bit of both.

Yet, I survived as thousands had before me in similar and worse conditions. Without a doubt, I was scarred for life; of that I was and still am sure. I endured nevertheless and held my head up high, in an attempt to mask my real persona: my total and helpless insecure bungling self, and extrovert to boot with no direction, only pseudo self-confidence. In any delicate, sensitive situation wherein I might be attacked verbally, physically, or mentally, naturally I would fold like a cheap suit, so help me. The micro-thin façade of phony self-confidence I portrayed was easily penetrated, easily dismantled. My life was rift with second guesses and the refusal to accept my lot in life, and to question myself into defeat however strong I was in character or physical strength. In other words, once I had a small fire at my feet, I would give up. Very childish, but that is where it all started. Of that I have accepted the truth and must not yet again fold.

Moving along with the story, I was now into the unfortunate throes of depression, strung out with acute severe anxiety, panic attacks, double vision, insomnia, diarrhea, mild bouts of paralysis, an inability to walk further than two blocks, an incredible pain in my right foot, specifically the arch, that was causing me to limp, possibly as a result of a ripped tendon, a pounding heart, and a fast pulse rate; and in all of this, everything was loud, double the volume, no triple the volume, essentially a deluge of noise nauseatingly high—yes, I know you're tired of hearing that, but it is true. I was continuing to lose weight, now down to 143 pounds from a robust weight for my height of 168; clothes and belts fit very loosely; there was a new development on my tongue, something akin to thrush, a red face, ears and neck, comparable to a niacin flush caused by an overload of nicotinic acid, lightheadedness that approached fainting, especially when sitting and trying to eat, a heavy pressing feeling on my chest, and intermittent bouts of constipation, most likely caused by Lexapro; I'd have to physically pull out grape-size balls of fecal matter less I blow out my ever-increasing hemorrhoids.

I suspect that all the straining that took place in about a two-week period forced right and left inguinal hernias or exacerbated preexisting conditions. I later had both repaired, again.

It took a mere twenty-four hours of Lexapro to flip my diarrhea to constipation, and this wasn't even planned for crying out loud. Perspiration kept flowing like a faucet not completely turned off, and there was no tomorrow, but I wished it would come; and I was unable to lower my constant, in-your-face fever which was a consequence of diverticulitis. A continuous fever is something no one should ever have, or it'll kill you by eventually frying your brain or by breaking down your organs, or both. Because of yet another allergy—this time to aspirin, which is mainly salicylic acid—I could not take it to lower my fever, and acetaminophens would touch off yet another bout of diarrhea. Aspirin caused me to break out in hives, while it simultaneously induced a mild asthma attack causing me to gasp for air until the drug wore off.

Hopelessly restless and experiencing a constant heavy pressure in my chest as if someone was sitting on me, accompanied with all the aforementioned, I returned to work, having enormous trouble typing letters, attempting to write emails, and just trying to calm my constant anxiety, and of what fear, I didn't know nor could I express. I couldn't speak to anyone without having to jump up and fly to the restroom. I had to urinate every half hour or so. I was in constant pain and severe anxiety from the tip of my graying hair to the bottom of my feet.

As I repeat, it was this constant need to go to the bathroom every thirty minutes, to either urinate, defecate, or both simultaneously, that further drove me to the brink of madness. I was never so completely out of control then with this abdominal disease and mental breakdown scenario, with no let-up in sight. By mid-February, I was suspended between being an emotional cripple and a totally mental wacko, if there's a separation of the two.

Continuing to lose weight, having chronic diarrhea, anxiety, and panic attacks were all accumulatively taking their toll on me, and my family doctor was at his medical "end of the rope" with what to do with me. Perhaps he had begun to question himself, much like I had. For example, on one visit, he asked me if he had prescribed Tequin, the antibiotic in pill form that set me off. He was relieved when I told him an emergency doctor had.

My doctor then said, "I've been treating you for over ten years. You've morphed into a delicate mental state that I'm not sure I can effectively treat. I may need to refer you to a psychiatrist." If he was thinking negative things about me, like this nutcase or whatever, it was not evident in his body language. He was sincere and sensitive in all respects; I couldn't ask for anything more. He then put me on an anxiety medicine Diazepam that proved ineffective after a few weeks, so he proceeded with 0.25 milligrams of Klonopin, a.k.a. Clonazepan, a benzodiazepine, a more potent and effective anti-anxiety and antipsychotic medicine. Of course, by now hearing me out thoroughly, and even though he had to move closer to hear me as I was now speaking in a very low and meek voice, he knew that he'd need to start me with a low dosage. The way with me, considering my age of sixty-three, became "start slow and start low," as in potency, but only after finding out the hard way with my incredibly overactive immune system. I didn't know if I was going to shit or go blind! Of all this, I knew that he had my best interests at heart. I was his patient, but also a friend with a common bond of science and astronomy.

Nevertheless, my mental health was continuing to deteriorate on a daily basis. "Bad to the bone" insomnia heightened my anxiety and kept me from recuperating. I was losing much sleep with the constant peeing, defecating, and high anxiety, which all had me twisting towels in my hands while writhing in discomfort from head to toe. Furthermore, I was experiencing numbness in my hands and feet during those many fretful nights which I came to dread. My hands and arms would have no feeling by the following morning and would only get back to normal by the end of the day. At night, every noise, including the normal soothing faraway toot of the night trains, sounded like it was in my room rumbling and blowing painfully in my ears. It appeared to me that the trains were rambling right through my upstairs guest bedroom, where I had to take up residence at night due to my severe erratic behavior. Even though the upstairs was carpeted, any pacing of the floor throughout the night would produce noise downstairs, so I tried in vain not to make a sound that could be heard. But I was as sick as a dog, so even no noise was a loud noise of silence anyway.

Such as it was, I couldn't turn down the volume of noise or stress in my head. It hurt me, and I couldn't do a damn thing about it but lie there and suffer. Everywhere I looked in that dark room, I saw a growing gloom that would envelope me with unbearable fear. It was like being back in Los Angeles, and I was a one-year-old child experiencing a nightmare. Double vision was keeping me so disoriented and dizzy to a point that I thought I'd shoot myself. I did have a handgun underneath my bed, waiting to blank me out of my misery.

Although I had some control, or so I thought, I was beginning to lose my grip with reality, slipping into a psychological black hole perhaps to never return, to then dwell eternally in some region between mental purgatory and a psychological hell; hell on Earth I was sure. I withdrew from all outside contact, from enjoyable activities and friends, even my mother, sister, and brother. I was sick; I guarantee you. To top it all, my beautiful dog, Tide, was suffering with prostate cancer as well as losing his hearing and vision and had become incontinent. Cataracts were heightening his inability to deal with moving around the house. His cancer was now giving him severe pain and severe anxiety, something you'd thought he learned from me. It was difficult to watch him deteriorate on an almost daily basis.

That February, bad Karma was descending on our house like a plague of ravenous locusts with no seagulls in sight. One morning while walking Tide, Diana tripped, fell, and broke her left arm, and I was of no use spiraling faster to a mental breakdown going nowhere. Painful panic attacks, anxiety, and palpitations were all running rampant in by mind and body, and I was about as useful as tits on a chicken to her. What's funny now is five years after my mental illness, I can recount my story as if I'm actually writing about someone else I knew back then. Perhaps, in that vein, I can reveal so much more that burrowed itself deeply into my physique, and like cream in a milk bottle floats to the top, my story too recently surfaced, if a little off chronologically. There's a tradeoff between remembering a painful event five years ago, telling it as an observer, but honestly, I have forgotten some issues or they became too deeply buried in my subconscious. Maybe I already said that. See what I mean?

With Diana's painful arm wrapped in ice, we spent a day at the emergency room with me like a loose cannon, or more like a spooked June bug flying erratically on a string. The emergency doctor X-rayed her arm and confirmed two broken bones in her left wrist. He wrapped her arm in a cast that started at her fingers and went all the way up to her armpit. Now she couldn't drive for twelve weeks and was severely restricted, and I wasn't so good myself, being fully nuts and all, hearing things up to three times their volume, and unable to focus on anything. By now, I was desperate.

I had spoken to my son-in-law, who had been an attendant in a mental ward, and asked him if he thought I was a candidate for the loony bin. He didn't know nor would he give me any recommendation. Somehow I now think that he may have thought that I was a couple of bricks shy of a full load, but he took me seriously and never once joked about my condition. How could I blame him for not discussing his father-in-law's mental instability? He spoke about the weird people he encountered while at one of North Carolina's mental institutions. Could I turn out to be one of those weirdoes too? By this time, being so flummoxed, I didn't know which way to turn; therefore, I decided to seek help again from my doctor.

He recommended that because my diverticulitis was now over six weeks old and counting, I should visit the gastroenterologist I'd seen back in 2000 when I had experienced a relatively short bout with that same disease. Again, he related that properly treated by competent doctors working as a team, they could lick my problems. Although my confidence in my health was "caca," he was positive and gave me the right vibes that would prove to be critical to my gradual improvement.

After a brief discussion with my gastroenterologist, he said, "The sulfa antibiotic should have knocked out your diverticulitis. I want you take Cipro. It's much easier on your system with fewer side effects than Tequin, yet it's similar in formulation. I'm prescribing you Cipro."

"But, doctor," I anxiously related, "it's another Fluoroquinolone, and I know I'll be allergic to it as well. I'm sure." He said in his usual calm bedside manner, "You're right, it is, but as I said earlier, it's a milder antibiotic less prone to the side effects of Tequin. You'll be okay taking it."

Reluctantly, my wife and I went to get the prescription that same afternoon. By 9:15 that night, I experienced a pulse rate of ninety-six; my heart was pounding, and my existing anxiety that had subsided some went into hyper drive. Right away, my wife phoned the gastroenterologist, while I was writhing in bed back up on the roller-coaster ride of being sick, pale, my heart pounding tremendously, and perspiring profusely. I was out of it yet again, but worse this time.

He said to her over the phone, "Okay, let's get him off Cipro and have him come to my office first thing in the morning."

The next morning, he saw me right away, gave me an examination, and said, "I'm prescribing Doxycycline and Flagyl. Take them for two weeks, come see me then, and I'm scheduling you for a colonoscopy on February 25." I concurred, felt somehow better, and I went home to take my drugs to get well. Mental exhaustion had me sleeping if I could during the day, and I can say that with the depression, the two left me lifeless, useless, and in a word, pathetic, a mere cardboard cutout of my real self. During this period, my sister called me wanting to fly over; she already had a round-trip ticket so that she could help us in our true time of need. Unfortunately, being off my rocker, I could hardly speak or think clearly, but I knew that I couldn't see her or anyone else, and the thought of it made me feel even worse. I was genuinely sick of body and mind, and Diana was in no position with her broken arm, and we had a very sick dog that was constantly bumping into our furniture. It was a veritable hell on Earth. I should mention, however, that if this had occurred even twenty years earlier, I'd have been institutionalized; no argument there.

A week later, I went back to see my gastroenterologist, as I was to fly out for an important corporate meeting in Chicago and needed his approval for the flight. I still had a fever, pain on my left side, and was now in continued full-blown anxiety with panic attacks, and right and left, I would hyperventilate at the least provocation, while my heart continuously pounded heavily in my chest. I could see the heart-pounding pulses in my eyes when I looked down at my feet or a white wall while urinating. That's how powerful my heartbeat was in that severe anxiety state.

The doctor approved my flight, but only after a very thorough rectal examination. Had he found prolepsis, or additional rectal infection, a consequence of an extended bout with diverticulitis; he said it would have meant a re-admittance to the hospital for surgery, and a round of yet more antibiotics, of what origin I could not have begun to imagine. I was beginning to feel like one giant swollen abdomen of anxiety and pain. He prescribed mega-sized suppositories to help combat any possible inflammation of the rectum. In other words, I was taking medicines orally and rectally now, burning the candle at both ends, so to speak. What could be more embarrassing?

19

Getting to the airport was no big issue, but having to go through the tightened security caused me yet more concern. A cardiologist I had been seeing in the interim because of irregular heartbeats—which I attributed to Tequin, an assumption that I couldn't take to the bank yet—put me on a one-month, shoulder heart monitor. My cardiologist calmed me with his bedside manner and thorough examination. One of the first questions I asked him after the exam was if I had had a heart attack or was I going to have one. He assured me that I was not going to have a heart attack, but to be on the safe side, he had me wear the monitor, especially considering my age. The chest unit with all the electrodes was menacing, if you can think of an octopus closely wrapped around your chest sucking out your bodily fluids.

Here's how I handled going through security, and the method was really stupid, but I was sick, you know, in a continuing descent into the Event Horizon of mental illness. Anyway, like an old macho man with an attitude, I yanked the monitor with the attached electrodes right off my chest and put the whole mess in one of the security bins. Knowing that I already had an allergy for the latex pads, the rip-off affect made the red bumps worse, so much worse, and with the numerous drugs coursing through my blood, I was "high man on cotton," or nearly delirious. Maybe that was the right way for me then in order to survive the long-running physical and mental ordeal that had started in early January. Anyone seeing me naked at that moment would have assumed without a doubt that a giant octopus had worked me over. The red patches had grown into nodules, but I made it to Chicago, nodules in drag and all.

Trying to have dinner at one of those fabulous Italian restaurants in Oakbrook that night with my associates in Chicago, I experienced overwhelming anxiety and panic attacks, constantly perspiring to "beat the band," while just right outside snow blanketed the parking lot where high winds and a temperature of twenty degrees Fahrenheit prevailed but offered me no relief or consolation. I knew going to Chicago was one, big crappy mistake, and it was already late February. Continuing to perspire profusely, I'd have to leave to go to the bathroom as if on some military agenda about every thirty minutes or so to relieve myself and dry off.

While wiping away profuse perspiration, I was so uncomfortable and having recurrent panic attacks. My cohorts finally took notice of my discomfort and asked me what they could do. This was dead-center winter in Chicago, and here I was sick as hell. I could have jumped off one of those tall Chicago buildings and not felt any pain; the only sure death would have been my salvation from this malady. Pure insanity was taking its toll on my body and brain! The meeting and dinner affair was over, and I got back to Charlotte, worse for wear, and my screwed up condition was holding firm. Furthermore, the suppositories I had to take to ward off the potential rectal dilemma were now becoming a real pain in the butt; this was true.

To my relief, the heart monitor did not confirm any permanent heart damage or irregularity. The technical term the cardiologist used failed me, but his letter assuaged some of my mounting anxieties concerning, specifically, my heart and circulatory system. My cardiologist, at every opportunity, assured me that I wasn't going to have a heart attack. Unfortunately, my disturbed and unstable mind thought differently, but I still kept his positive attitude close to my heart; no pun intended. Truth be told, in my mind, I had wanted an ironclad assurance with guarantees. But there are none in the medical field ever.

Getting back to my gastroenterologist, he scheduled an MRI of my abdomen, as I was having cramps and more pain, and he suspected that the sacs in my left abdomen might distend further, ultimately exploding, and like an appendicitis, would result in painful death if not caught early. My whole damn body was fraught with potentially fatal consequences, and mentally, I wasn't feeling so good myself. A friend of mine earlier on had lost his father to diverticulitis, and this was foremost in my mind. I now knew that diverticulitis was no disease to fool around with. Whether I would survive this ordeal was anyone's guess.

Unfortunately, the evening I was to have my MRI, those unpredictable panic attacks crippled me. To say I was red to the bone in color was to state the obvious. I should have never driven to the hospital by myself, but Diana was at home way too encumbered with her arm in a cast to have driven me. I was on my sick-ass own! The nurses and technicians contacted the gastroenterologist to determine what to do. Additional Klonopin, over 1.5 milligrams, was prescribed, a very high dosage for me. They waited a half an hour for me to calm down. The extra medication really didn't help, but it allowed me sufficient time to get my breath back so I could go through the test. I still felt like hell, and my heart and head felt like they would burst. What a ball of crap!

Although he found no complications, I was to return the next day for more tests. What may have contributed to the panic attack prior to the MRI scan was an accident I had had two nights earlier. While taking some recycle items to the trash bin at night, I tripped on my firewood stack and cut my left ankle. I suffered tremendous mental anguish over a relatively simple wound. In my mental condition, having little reason or focus, I thought the wound would never heal. Had I also developed diabetes since the wound would not heal? I questioned my every thought and mood. I didn't have diabetes, but I assumed I did. With my blood sugar distorted by Tequin, who in the hell would know? Not realizing that the ankle area has relatively low blood flow, the wound naturally took weeks to heal. I hadn't figured that out or thought that through at that point. The cut and pain on top of everything else drove me further down the dark path of insanity. You didn't want to know me then. Would I become a virtual recluse? Only time would tell.

An unscheduled trip to the headquarters of one of my main customers came up, and even though I was so sick, I had to go, less earlier efforts for new business were compromised. This time I didn't discuss it with any of my doctors; I just went. Fuck it! Going into Terre Haute, Indiana, was not a big deal, but I was hopelessly anxious. In a conversation a week later, a friend told my wife that his girlfriend had seen me at the Charlotte airport, and that I looked gaunt, ashen-faced, and very sick. I knew this to be true. The customer meeting went without conflict, and it actually went smoothly. I was able to nail down one of their new facilities. But after finishing business and while at the airport, I began having anxiety issues for no apparent reason. Waiting at the gate, a horrible panic attack hit me with a vengeance, and I took my anxiety pills like M&Ms, but to no avail. It was so bad on the plane that a doctor on board came to my assistance, told me to massage my vagus nerve, which is on the left side of the neck, and had me breathe into a paper bag. When I arrived into Charlotte, the stewardess requested a wheelchair for me; however, I was feeling better by then and thanked her and got into my car, and finally to the comfort of my home. I didn't have the strength to go to work the next day, but I did the remainder of the week, although still feeling sick as hell.

The next week, I went in for the dreaded colonoscopy. The preparation to clean out my colon thoroughly threw me into another panic attack. These attacks were seemingly eating at my innards, but no one knew. I was the Lone Ranger on this deal.

The attending nurse assisting my doctor, said, "My God, Bob, your arms and legs are so cold. Should I say, cold hands, warm heart?" Embarrassed over my mental condition, I held my tongue and thoughts to myself. Deep depression, extreme anxiety, loss of weight, and being clammy may have been the causes for my cold body. Was I in cold storage yet? When the doctor came in to start the procedure, I told him that Lipitor was regulating me and that I should stop taking Citrucel to increase my fiber content. I might have that wrong, though; maybe I said that Citrucel now had me regulated, and I should stop taking Lipitor. Well, whatever, I still take Lipitor today, strictly to lower my cholesterol and triglycerides. I get most of my daily fiber from cereals, fruits, and vegetables. Those eight glasses of water per day keep me hydrated too, and the water count is one thing I constantly keep track of in my head. Now is that crazy or what?

The colonoscopy turned out to confirm diverticulitis, but nothing else, and I was cleared of any cancerous polyps.

Through all the tedium of pain, fever, ill health, and anxiety, I was taking more medicines than I could manage, and I called several of my doctors insisting they tell me what was contraindicated and what was allowed before a negative reaction would occur. Two were particularly helpful, my internist and the neurologist. (I will cover the neurologist in a later chapter.) But even after confirming what I should or shouldn't do with the pills from what their nurses told me, I would get mixed up. This going back and forth irritated me. I was curious to know what they thought of me.

Armed with some advice from the doctors and nurses and my limited knowledge of drugs—I had two *Physician's Desk References* in my library at the time, but they were outdated—I made a grid on a three-by-five-inch index card and kept thorough records of when I took the medicines and the dates, the times, and potency. As a couple of days passed, keeping the record and taking the medicines became an obsession that got definitely out of hand. I dreamed, talked, and bored my wife and sister and others with what seemed like a tedious overindulgence and the outrageous time I took keeping the cards and records straight. Undoubtedly, this was a meaningless obsession. What was it all about? Did I think I was a pharmacist required to keep meticulous records in compliance with the FDA, OSHA, or another government regulation? Did the FBI keep tabs on my medicines, frequency of use, and when I took them? Were they going to burst in any minute and confiscate all my stuff? Hell no, I didn't want them messing with my stuff! This was my mental illness and no one else's. What's strange is in all my stupor and depression, you'd think I would cry for hours; I mean, just bawl my eyes out. Well, no, and I didn't know why. For whatever reason, no tears welled up in my eyes the entire time I was in a state of depression, but I could have shot myself instead.

I'm sure you would have wanted to see my index cards, because they were madly scribbled with more lines between lines, as I was trying to conserve paper, with font size so small even I had trouble making out my small grade-school-looking handwriting. There's no matrix that I can think of that matched the hyper-ridiculousness of my cards. What a stupid joke my mind played on me! Maybe it's important to review just how many prescribed medicines I was into then. I was taking all of the following several times a day or in combination along with a few supplements: Klonopin, Ambien, Valium then Xanax, Lexapro then Celexa, Lipitor, Citrucil for fiber, Doxycycline, Flagyl, vitamins and Hydroxyzone, and Tylenol with codeine for pain. There were supplements such as Ensure, vitamins, and other drugs, alas some of which I have since forgotten. To say that the aforementioned meds were an inconsequential cocktail shotgun approach to cure me would be a disservice. They were prescribed on an individual and/or combination basis to get me well quickly. That much I firmly believed. Let me also say that I was astounded at the coolness and professional manner in which the doctors and nurses received my incessant phone calls and frequent questionings about the medicines I was taking. If not available, they'd get back to me with answers concerning how each medicine may have been contraindicated if taken out of order, together, late, or not at all. With little to no medication-management skills and less knowledge with these new pharmaceuticals, I had to rely totally on the information they gave me or the literature therein contained when prescriptions were filled. Their confidence in relaying information to me with a workable medicine schedule was reassuring.

One possible area of potential conflict was the frequent doctor visits I needed to have in order to stay on track with progress, the tests, medications, and supposed improvement. I made yet another grid for the vast amount of doctors and appointment dates. I don't remember missing any of the appointments, but it was damn hard to keep them straight in light of my mental confusion and instability, all in the bloom of psychosis. So there I was effectively mired in updating two index cards every day for two independent issues and me certifiably "out to lunch." Suffice to say that visiting those doctors recommended and who I felt could help me was a testament to my unashamed eagerness to get well and put the embarrassment of mental illness quickly behind me. Could you blame me? If I were running in circles with professionals in academia, they would have dropped me like a hot potato if they had an inkling of my dilemma with mental illness. I can't say that I would have blamed them either.

In my constant visits and travel to and from my doctors' offices, and there were too many to list, my family doctor and I agreed that I should be put on short-term disability. I was going nowhere fast in reverse with this horrible condition, and the mere thought of driving, flying, or making a marketing presentation were giving me thoughts of a quick end to it all. I couldn't face the world anymore. Maybe I was being punished for my past indiscretions with women, friends, and others you would be bored for me to list. You see, I never clearly remember from my younger days whether I had slept with six women in seven days or seven women in six days, or if I even called any of them back; such was the habit of my inconsiderate, selfish, and immature self. So, there I was fucked up, and my good karma had disintegrated right there and then, as I had nothing of ethereal value to offer the karma gods in return. This was no quid pro quo to affect a reasonable or equitable exchange.

Just before going on short-term disability, one of my cohorts, a lovely lady whom I had privately lusted after and who worked in quality control, asked if she could see me. Knowing that I had now been sick for several weeks and looked like death warmed over, she mentioned that I should start eating yogurt right away and even recommended a brand that contained a small amount of fiber to help me with the alimentary canal issue. Her recommendation was to eat at least a cup of yogurt a day, an excellent suggestion, although I loathed yogurt then and perceived it as an unnecessary supplement. Anyhow, not discounting her suggestion, that evening I started on yogurt, fortified with a protein and vitamin supplement, as suggested by the psychologist I was seeing. My weight now being 143, I suffered from a white-coated tongue, daily panic and anxiety attacks, lingering diverticulitis, little to no sleep, and suicidal tendencies, and I nearly conceded in my mind that I was finally ready for the "big bin." Judging, however, with a paranoid mind, I also felt my doctor may have been ready to get me off his case, as I had become more than he could handle, and in the way, a pest. Make no mistake, though, he was on my side with my best interests at heart. Rest assured, there's no argument, but no denying it too, I was fucked up in so many ways.

Chapter 4

Along the Way, I Lost My Mind and Needed Help

My internist, by now proving to be a very skilled clinician yet able to reconcile that he could not handle my escalating mental problems, decided that I needed another doctor who specialized in handling someone going "bonkers." He didn't say that, but I knew, nevertheless. Though he insisted that I see a psychiatrist, I shuttered and went clammy with perspiration at the possibility of having that stigma, and I was embarrassed at the thought, that is, having been referred to a head doctor. This was now surely the last straw for me. In my delusions, you can appreciate how I didn't think I was sick enough to see such a doctor. So under duress from me, he decided that the best course for my treatment would be to refer me to a clinical psychologist who was very experienced in the field of depression and anxiety. I had met my doctor half way, a nice compromise. The psychologist he recommended turned out to be the best foot forward in the battle to normalcy, and I was one of her preferred patients, if that were even possible in a doctor—patient scenario.

By early March, as the Doxycycline and Flagyl had finally put that damn diverticulitis that lasted for over ten weeks to bed, I started seeing the psychologist twice a week because Tequin had stripped away all my physical strength and left me in a critical mental state with volumes of anxiety. Was I a mass of crap potentially ready to blow, or had I been like that all along? You can bet being on short-term disability saved me from further embarrassment with my friends and coworkers. I couldn't face the public anymore. My difficulties centered on my extreme anxiety, panic attacks, insomnia, frequent urination and defecation, loss of concentration, and the absolute need to sleep during the day. Hell, I wasn't sleeping at night; how would this end? I was so nervous by then to the point of derangement. The thought of permanent psychosis further depressed me, and I could think of nothing else, not even sex for crying out loud.

Deep depression brought the worst out in me. Mental paralysis resigned me to a mild case of catatonia. Oh, was I ever paralyzed by paranoia and extreme irrational fear! For what fear or caution I never knew or found out. I went dark in no time flat! I could no longer sleep or dream. I saw the end coming with every minute of the day ticking constantly all the way and especially throughout the night. I feared the night with unbearable dread. I didn't want to live this way anymore and loathed leaving the house. Diana said one day, "You have developed the dull, glazed look of someone perhaps on barbiturates. On second thought, more like one who has just finished a big dinner and is ready for a nap. Which are you, Bob?" Of course, I couldn't respond.

I was caught in limbo with a physical body, saddled with the mind of a ghost, living in a time right before death, one foot in the grave while the other on ice, and I was unforgivingly bushwhacked by my own dark mind. Had my gray matter turned to dark matter, and was I now in the event horizon of a mental black hole of hell?

I was given to short-term catatonic stupors, sitting in a corner chair for hours not saying a thing, just staring blankly, transfixed on nothing. I stayed at home physically and mentally exhausted, drained of my once beautiful and eloquent self, or so I thought. No more could I speak, not even for the length of a minute, and forget my mojo, my sexual self however strong had also tumbled out of my life, perhaps never to be regained. I figured my dried arrangement was destined to never bloom again and to be unemployed for the rest of its existence. It was double jeopardy for me, at home not working mentally or physically. There was no optimism to cling to; I was done in. Even my "radio mouth" had evaporated to a whisper to short, staccato phrases. Several friends, if you can call them that, referred to me as a "radio" because they perceived me as talking continuously, and most of them were as guilty as I was of the same damn thing, perhaps worse in some cases. Walking for a mere two blocks was such an agonizing and painful experience that I stopped trying. My legs, especially my calves, felt like two cinder blocks holding me back with noticeable pain. I don't quite remember everything, but those are things that distinctly fill my memory of illness, or so I have been told. I do have my memory, however vague. Cobweb memories festooned with dust like particles connect me loosely to those days, and I have to wrack my brain to remember even one iota and think carefully how it was then.

It is difficult now to pursue and arrange chronologically those events that happened over five years ago in a sensible and effective manner. Did I embellish my condition then or now, or was it gospel then? I'm told it was very bad. The truth didn't set me free then and not now, nor has any of the pain endured in that time period left me for one moment. The pain is there, if only now intertwined in the memory of a partial amnesiac. In other words, the pain and whatever memory of that six-month period is in part sequestered in my subconscious. Thinking through the whole damn mess could be my undoing. It's as if I must relive and experience that horrible time in order to relate the story correctly.

My mother, living in San Antonio and never having to witness my stupor, anxiety, and most ridiculous condition, recognized the pain and discomfort I was going through and sent me a "get well" card twice a week. She didn't have much money, so I asked her not to send me so many cards, but she refused. She told me the cards only cost her fifty cents each, and it was no burden on her. Actually, truth be told, I secretly loved her doing that. It was some consolation to me, especially the sacrifice she made. I wasn't even worth it, but apparently she thought differently. My self-esteem had hung out to dry for some time now, but it lifted with each card I received from her. She was always my biggest fan. She also sent me those incredible short inspirational books that in retrospect provided me a lot of comfort. I have to admit they really helped me. I do realize this now, if not then, in that paranoid state of depression, confusion, and uncertainty. You need to understand that she had already been through two open-heart surgeries, a carotid artery surgery, a bladder reversal, and a tumor was removed from her throat, all over several decades, and she came through with such a positive attitude. No person should have had to endure such suffering and pain, but she did so with flying colors.

Here I was in those interminable pains of mental anguish and hell. Why hadn't she suffered depression or anxiety like I experienced? Was I some inconsequential wuss? Why me? Did I inherit a dysfunctional mental gene from my father's side of the family? My parents separated shortly after I was born. Was I to go through life blaming myself for their eventual divorce? That entire situation may have affected my young mind and set the stage for my future mental quandaries.

Nevertheless, my fault or not, in this illness I became more withdrawn, mentally blank, annoyingly insecure, and endlessly asked the same questions over and over. Claustrophobia may have been yet another phobia overwhelming me.

Without thinking through the process or any mental screening on my part, I'd say to Diana, and do remember embarrassingly, "Should I call work and tell them when I'll return? Is it okay for me to state my condition to my boss or my coworkers? Maybe I shouldn't say anything about my mental state? Surely they'll fire me. Don't you agree? Should I call the doctor? Should I call John?" Now you'd think that I did this just once or twice the entire time. On the contrary, I did this many times hourly and daily, not even remembering or caring what I'd said earlier. I was an open faucet of verbal vomit propelling effusively onto anyone within earshot, and I repeated myself constantly. My obsessive, continuous blathering of nervous questions became the mainstay of my conversations, and for Diana, they were hopelessly one-sided and fruitless, for sure meaningless. Weren't they the rantings of a whacked out, poor soul? She didn't patronize me though. Of the small link to reality, I knew instinctively that she was sincere. Yet, I have to admit that our conversations—that is, when I spoke—were then mere nonsequiturs, as I really couldn't relate to anything directly verbal. Truthfully, I struggled to communicate effectively, and under the circumstances that was an enormous task for me wherein I failed miserably.

This constant questioning and pain-in-the-ass insecurity went on and on with no apparent end in sight. Suffice to say, I was in a knife-edge state of high anxiety with several medicines trying unsuccessfully to calm me down and return me to a state of normalcy. In that delirious state, I had come to stabilize, if that is remotely possible, to some place between almost insane to basically insane. Diana, holding her own but straining at the seams, was beginning to lose her patience with me.

How could I blame her? She noticed another change in me, and it was that my infectious smile had disappeared. A scowl had replaced that ubiquitous smile. Permanent lines of pain furrowed my once line-free face.

Eating at home or at a restaurant became rather impossible. It was a predictable chore and a source of unbelievable conflict for us. I picked at everything; it all seemed so repulsive to me. I couldn't stay seated for more than ten to fifteen minutes without my vision tunneling where I would nearly pass out. If I didn't stand up, go to the bathroom, of which I was doing all the time anyhow, or go to Diana's car, I knew I would faint or self-combust; there was no way around it. Furthermore, I suspected that most of the food served to me was contaminated, toxic, or filled with hair, worms, or garbage. It was garbage all the way down. The water, tea, and juices served to me became a target of my revulsion, likewise with food in general. Actually, I stopped drinking all kinds of tea and all sodas that first week in January after I had noticed a decided elevation of my heart pounding and a constant pulsing in my eyesight and realized it was directly related to the caffeine in those kinds of drinks while taking the antibiotic. This was confirmed in the pharmaceutical literature on Tequin that caffeine could heighten the strength of the medicine I was prescribed.

To this day, I drink neither tea nor sodas; it's mostly water for me and only 100 percent fruit juices. I usually extend the juices with about 25 percent Brita-filtered water and have decided to up that to 35 percent to help lower the sugar content. No freely added sugar is mixed with the 100 percent fruit juice drinks, but I still want to lower my sugar intake, be it simple or complex sugars. This does leave me some room to eat dark chocolate, one bad habit I have had consistent trouble eliminating. If you wonder whether I'm paranoid about food today, I am with some but not to the extent experienced while in that state of being "flipped."

I have occasional tunneling of vision today, and it generally goes away; however, if I see any constellations that's only because I may be studying the night skies. I attribute the infrequent tunneling today to a comparatively low blood pressure that is usually in the 110/60 range, pulse rate of 52 to 60, maybe a little low, but still not bad for a part-time hiker, not to mention a senior citizen.

By early April 2005, my visits to the psychologist were reduced to once a week, mainly because she was not seeing sufficient improvement in my mental state. It is possible that I had a biochemical instability that could only be corrected by medicines—a realignment of my brain chemicals was definitely a necessity to get me back to being normal—and she could not prescribe drugs; only a medical doctor could. However, while treating me, if she thought it necessary, she would confer with my family doctor to increase, diminish, or change my dosage to a different prescription based on my progress or lack of it, but apparently this was insufficient. In all fairness to her, she never used any psychobabble with me. No, it was straight to the cause without any esoteric hogwash or superfluous chitchat. When I consider that period, she may have felt my time with her was up, and subsequently, that I might fare better with a psychiatrist. And no, there were no subtle shifts in her perspective of me. She was straight arrow, no shitting me.

I remember sharing with her in March that I felt my career with my company was over, as I could not bear to face the public, give presentations, or ever fly again. She explored this and discussed those issues in depth with me. Her positive manner with me went a long way in helping me to restore some of my lost confidence and sanity. If she thought so, she never alluded to my being a candidate for the loony bin, either. She never called me a psycho-ceramic, i.e., a crackpot, either. One point on her sincerity is when we exchanged concerns about Lipitor, one of the statins of choice to reduce cholesterol. I was taking a five-milligram pill every other day, and she was taking forty milligrams daily. For her size and age, and considering that she was only about five foot two, maybe 120 pounds, and around fifty-two years of age, I felt it was too high a dosage and thought my small contribution might help in some way. What's more, her initial cholesterol was actually lower than my initial number. Whether she discussed lowering the potency with her doctor, I never found out, but I hope she did.

Assured of her expertise in therapy and professional manner, I would have recommended her to Rasputin, Ted Kaczynski, or Charles Manson, and she may have rehabilitated them all, guaranteed. She was that good. But medicines were critical here not behavior, or strictly counseling on a one-to-one therapeutic basis. Furthermore, without proper medication to relieve my depression and anxiety, something more in keeping with the work of a psychiatrist, I would have continued to relentlessly question my every thought, movement, and action until the universe would collapse in one big crunch. In light of so much mental confusion, indecision, questioning, and inability to work through the simplest of scenarios, it's no wonder temporary mental paralysis arose so dramatically in me. Unquestionably, more medical help and the correct one was desperately needed if restored sanity was the ultimate goal. It was. I have often wondered and thought that Tequin may have tapped into the portion of my brain that contained an already fragile mind, wherein all those weird and upsetting things I harbored lay ready to surface. In other words, Tequin may have significantly magnified my potential preexisting mental aberrations. Who knew?

Chapter 5

A Journey to the Unknown or They've Come to Take Me Away

While awaking from a particularly hellish nightmare one morning, I felt someone slowly pushing me through a dimly lit hall. It's as if I was floating in time and space in slow motion. Immediately realizing I was sitting in a wheelchair and noticing that all attendants were dressed in white uniforms, I knew I was in a hospital or a mental institution. Here the rooms had only one unshaded bulb lighting each room, and people drifted aimlessly throughout the halls dragging their tattered urine-saturated clothes and walking through the halls half naked. No doubt about it, I had been committed and my biggest fear realized. This place reeked of lunacy and death, a mental ward after all with a Dostoyevskian twist. Most wandering patients had rough, dry skin that covered mere bones giving a withered, gaunt look. Several wore beat-up shoes with holes and soles that flapped like clogging shoes. But here they danced to an entirely different beat, one originating only in their minds. Many men, not having shaved for months, displayed long, unkempt beards. Their dull, dilated eyes showed blankly, while their bodies gave off the putrid stench of death, and maybe they *were* dead.

This was not a military establishment, but a pill-popping, dirty institution, a veritable nuthouse any way you could cut it. Who committed me here? How was it Diana had not intervened just like she had for me in my second emergency visit earlier in that year when I still had it pretty much together? Why was I here in view of my greatest, absolutely most frightening obsession that I had harbored? Had I, in some state of confusion, committed myself unknowingly and just couldn't remember? Was this a deep-down need for attention, a push and pull in my mind much like the struggle of the sea intertwined with the moon, only I was intertwined with myself? In my left arm an IV fed me some drug that I could only make out as "Te," the rest of the word escaping me. Oh, shit! It dawned on me! Someone had forced me to take Tequin again. Oh, God! Where was that emergency doctor? I bet she was behind this whole bloody mess and back on my case.

Who was pushing my wheelchair? I turned around to see who it might be and discovered it was that psychiatrist who had so blatantly passed me off as a raving lunatic, and to him I may have been, but because he wanted to retire soon, he had no desire to take me on as a patient. To him, I was a nuisance, way too complicated, so far gone and zonked out the yin-yang and too far off the charts for any rehabilitation. As his patient, he would have immediately committed me to this ward, sequestering me for infinity, to the dreaded mental black hole of hell I had dreamed of on several occasions. Maybe he was some half-assed celebrity for all I knew. I later thought him as sympathetic as a hooded man about to cleave one's head right off. You may know the type!

As he wheeled me through the long hallway, I could see patients in rooms being whacked on their backs, as if in some archaic spirit removal fashion, for reasons I could not imagine. In another room, a woman obliviously rubbed her center of sexual pleasure while a nurse flogged her repeatedly at about the same speed culminating in a convulsion of satisfaction rather than pain on the patient's face. She must have been mentally and physically abused as a child to the extent that she needed that kind of punishment, a form of penitential retribution to calm her wild spirit and satisfy her sexual need. In another room, there sat a person who was tightly hugging his meager belongings held in a poorly sewn-up burlap bag, all the while mumbling nonsensibly. No one gave him the time of day. In another room, a wily-haired doctor operated on a patient as he removed something from a woman's abdomen that I couldn't make out to positively identify. Could have been a baby or a tumor, who knows? Another patient was undergoing a lobotomy for sure, or what was that long ice pick-like instrument in his hand, and so many surgical tools lying askew on a dirty gurney? Was that a partial brain laying on the other empty gurney? This was unbelievable, a nightmare from hell!

What was happening, and where was I? Who was going to win the battle raging in my lugubrious, twisted mind, the Germans or the Russians? The Spanish or the Americans? Napoleon? Whoever won would lose the battle for want of a nail, a shoe, a horse, a rider, and the kingdom, and in this case, my sanity, even my life, as I had known it for Christ's sake. Had I met my Waterloo? "Lions and tigers and bears, oh my!"

I started to struggle in my wheelchair trying to stand up, and then it dawned on me that both of my arms were bound behind my back. When I looked down I noticed that I had on a white jacket, actually a straightjacket. So really I had been taken away. That son of a bitch had run me in after all.

Just as fast as this whole scenario was playing out, I awoke with a start. Everything disappeared right before me for no apparent reason. What really happened? The images had been hallucinations created in my subconscious wherein I had little control, and they were projected onto my imaginary mental screen. It was pure nonsense, created by an inebriated-by-drugs mind. Suddenly with a whole-body seizure that occurred for only a split second, my Chippendale leather chair materialized as I realized I had been sitting on it mentally frozen in time for what seemed like several days, in a catatonic state with a blank look, focusing on nothing that I could remember and seeing through cataract-developing, dilated pupils. Later I was told that often I sat on the living room chair staring into space, not speaking or moving for days. I could ascribe this fake prestidigitation swindle of a mind still burning from the residual, toxic drug Tequin, which I'm sure as hell was the reason for temporarily going off my rocker. There was no other plausible explanation. Would this haunt me for months or years to come? Tequin was largely responsible; I'm sure. I didn't just make up the whole screwed-up story, nor could I attribute the craziness to my parents or grandparents or cast any aspersions on my ancestry. They never showed any outward appearance of being mentally ill. It should be stressed that I've never been that clever or knowledgeable of mental patients to conjure up such a convoluted mental story with all the accoutrements. Do you think I made this shit up? Hell no! And I'm not some inconsequential crybaby or whiner. I was physically sick first, then mentally, for crying out loud.

Developing mental illness in the final stretch of one's life usually doesn't just occur by happenstance, that is, without some valid reason. There's a cause and effect, by God, or I may have to whip somebody's ass to get to the bottom of this illness. Anyhow, you choose! There may have been someone out there who knew about these things. I sure as hell didn't.

So I ramble on and digress; let me get back to the story. Another theory that could explain how I came to be in the unbelievable high-anxiety state was that Tequin somehow severed the control gate of flight-or-fright adrenalin regulation of my adrenal cortex. The adrenal glands secrete adrenaline throughout the nervous system when specifically needed. In my case, adrenalin was entirely too free flowing whether I was awake or asleep. I slept very little and wondered throughout the upstairs rooms desperately seeking sleep, and that went on for months. The neurological distress caused by a rampant flow of adrenalin threw me into a 24/7 frazzle. I couldn't connect the dots between reality and fantasy and relax for even a minute. I was on edge the entire time. The medicines prescribed to counter Tequin worked marginally, but they were a logical start. Mental therapy wasn't working, but at least I had a professional audience with which to start some sort of rehabilitation, albeit sporadic at first.

Having now been continuously using antibiotics of different origins since January 5 with no apparent end in sight, in addition to of all the existing conditions, I developed a white, thick coating on my tongue. The white tongue threw me into yet another series of panic attacks. How many panic attacks could any human endure without going deeper into the darker shadows of a full-blown psychosis?

Anyhow, I went to see my dentist, and while having my teeth cleaned, I experienced yet another confounded and unbelievable panic attack. Why did I now have another panic attack, especially in a rather benign environment? I didn't know. Luckily, the dental assistant, a young woman in her late twenties, noticed my problem and came to my rescue. She mentioned that she had been having panic attacks for a couple of years, and she was only in her twenties. Although then it didn't seem to help me much, her describing her condition, in retrospect, I know it did. Misery loves company, as pundits say, so we had ourselves a mutual problem. She advised me right there and then how to soften the attacks, but I'm sure I passed her advice off as inconsequential. What she recommended was to breathe deeply and slowly until a calm came over me.

After a quick examination, my dentist said that what I had was not thrush, but a condition as a result of overuse of antibiotics, and he recommended an instrument with which one could scrape off the white coating. This helped physically, but it didn't address the cause of the coating. Scraping off the coating was only superficial, and it would return after a couple of hours. My dentist asked why my face was so flushed and red. I couldn't really answer him correctly or directly and evaded the question as best as I could. I didn't know what caused my red, flushed face that was much like a niacin flush from an overdose of that vitamin, but I had it for several months while experiencing the anxiety and panic attacks, and it was definitely not a result of niacin. I wasn't taking it then.

Getting back to the white coating on my tongue and other intestinal issues, my gastroenterologist recommended probiotics. I took them quickly as yogurt by itself had not diminished the coating or the stomach cramps. Probiotics and regular yogurt eventually regulated and squared away my white coating and my diarrhea to an extent.

Although the Lexapro had me constipated, it had done little to relieve some of my other inconvenient discomforts already discussed, mainly anxiety, mounting phobias, and depression, especially depression. It may have been that I had not been taking it for a sufficient amount of time.

How I perceived psychology, i.e., the treatment of mental disorders, up to that time in 2005 was simple. Mental disorders to me appeared as concentric circles, much like when a stone hits a pond. The mental disorder closest to the point of the stone's entry was usually the hardest to diagnose, as it was more nearly normal, while mental disorders at the outermost circle were easiest to label, diagnose, and eventually treat. If you can't clearly identify the disorder, how can you treat it? Well, that's why the shotgun approach using a general antipsychotic drug oftentimes is prescribed, hoping to net and successfully treat the malady.

What must happen next to get me healthy and back to work? God dammed, I didn't want to be institutionalized.

Chapter 6

Mind the Gap

By mid-March, I was pretty much over diverticulitis and my white-coated tongue. A very low-grade fever remained as a reminder of the ordeal. But with the fever, random tunneling vision, anxiety, irregular heartbeats, panic attacks, and the aforementioned maladies coming to the forefront, it could all be described in one file titled mental illness. Its precise name is not important. Were those anxiety and panic attack issues precipitated by Tequin, or were they always there sequestered in my consciousness, or really simply mental imperfections resuscitated by Tequin? I know I've said this before, but it was Tequin that did me in! No one can refute that in good conscience. Yes, I had been given to a lack of confidence, light anxiety, and self-doubt in my youth as a result of the uncommon events of growing up penniless and fatherless, reared by a mother who worked herself to the bone and was hardly ever there due to her fifty-hour long work weeks. But what really did it to me then was an improperly vetted drug.

My eyes never exhibited a total lapse from reality, although some may have disagreed; yet, I still couldn't focus on anything tangible that might give me or my wife a sense of improvement. Knowing Tequin made me mentally sick unfortunately did nothing to help me get well. To say I resembled and walked like a zombie might be closer to the truth then, and yet I was so supersaturated with anxiety that the mental weight could have caused me to fall through the center of the Earth like an ounce of material from a white dwarf. Why was I so off balance like a ship listing to one side laden with water?

In that state one day, I found that I couldn't stand up straight, was constantly dizzy, and my heart raced uncontrollably. Now starting to recognize that I finally had bought the farm, Diana dropped me off at the emergency room wanting little part of my sickness. No, she wasn't so much put out by my illness as much as she thought that I might be faking it, if that was even possible. Could I blame her? She was enduring two very painful situations plus mine. As mentioned before, Tide, our Boston terrier, was suffering from prostate cancer, white-eyed with cataracts and deaf. To further cause him pain, the fluoroquinolone antibiotic he was prescribed at that time caused him to have seizures. He'd walk a little, fall as a result of unconsciousness, suffer a seizure, and then regain consciousness a bit later. Prior to the antibiotic, he never suffered a seizure. The other issue that Diana dealt with simultaneously was the pain and discomfort of her left total-arm cast. The cast immobilized her from getting anything done, and she lost weight from both issues and certainly from my constant illness, too.

Another experience with Tide happened late one evening. While walking around the house in great pain, he got entangled in some computer and telephone wires next to our bed. As I tried to extricate him from all the wires, he inadvertently bit my left thumb—that's pretty good since he was blind—and blood spurted out and only stopped about thirty minutes later after applying pressure to the mangled thumb. The next morning, my doctor's nurse confirmed that I would not need a tetanus shot. Those shots are good for ten years, and the previous year I had been given a booster. Tide went on later that year to get much worse, as was expected considering he was now well into his fifteenth year. Upon recommendation from our veterinarian, we put him to sleep. Diana cried for a month over our sweet, lovable dog, an angel on Earth. He went to his death so stoic and innocent that I cried too like a baby with severe colic. Today, we still miss him so much. He was the most respectful dog that ever walked this Earth.

At the hospital, the emergency attending male nurse, the same one from my very first visit in early January for diverticulitis, gave me little attention, took the basic vitals, and left town in my mind. This nurse would not answer any of my questions, would not let me see any of the blood tests taken including liver enzymes and so forth, and in all refused to give me the time needed to explain my condition. Unmoved by my continued requests, he even refused to have the attending physician see me. Perhaps the two were laughing their butts off, exchanging hand slaps, jokes, and otherwise having a great time over my illness. I had gone to emergency because I was sick and desperate to get well, not pretending to be sick. The hospital never reconciled that Tequin caused my mental illness. They just kept charging me for every pill, test, or time spent at the hospital that was not as a result of diverticulitis. The only hospital visit that should have been on my account or insurance company's account was the first visit. The other two should have been on the hospital's tab.

They kept me overnight for observation. I glanced at the wall clock in my room that read 11:28 p.m., took off my glasses, and dozed off. It couldn't have been more than five minutes when a young nurse kissed me on the cheek and then my mouth while groping me, and I gasped not knowing what to do. Her cleavage left me little room for imagination, and I found myself coming to life. She said, "Someone asked me to come in here and make you happy because you were so down, but I can easily see you're up, way up. Are you feeling better? " I was speechless. She bent over to pick up a magazine, and that's when I realized she was naked underneath her candy stripe dress, or whatever she wore. What was this lovely lady doing with an old coot like me? I asked her if the real nurse knew she was in here and where security was. The security thing bothered me, because if we were going to do anything, I wanted some privacy and didn't want anyone barging in on us in some uncompromising position. She shook her head and didn't answer me, but then started to grope me again. I sensed something was very wrong. At that instant, I felt dizzy, confused, and very light-headed. And then, startled, I woke up, and the clock marked 11:32 p.m. Only four minutes had passed. I had dreamed the whole affair! How unfortunate? Why hadn't I stayed asleep? It was a lot nicer seeing her in my dreams.

Early the next morning, I was released without as much as a visit or word from the emergency care doctor or the male nurse. In other words, I had been on my own; I felt this deep down to my bones and hoped this was not to be the medical care of the future. Because I insisted that my condition resulted from Tequin made me someone they needed to get rid of as soon as possible. I left with, "Don't let the door hit you in the ass when you leave, or for God's sake don't come back." What a bunch of crap! The visit had been a waste of their time and money, and apparently mine and my insurance company's as well. I felt cheated, as I should have. The horny dream is all I walked away with from the hospital ordeal.

This brings to mind something in my immediate illness that I've had to deal with, and that is the thought of death. At every significant peak of illness where the outcome was suspect, that is, where I might pass on, I felt there had been déjà vu; maybe I had somehow in my mind prepared for the inevitable. Could it be that illness is a preparation for death? Are we conditioned to secretly think it? Well, I don't know or think so. Though millions do die as a result of an illness, however long or short in duration, accidents, or from complications of any kind of surgery be it minor or major. Is death the final stage of any protracted illness, as it seems to me?

Every time my vision tunneled and I was headed for the floor, I would bolt and fight the darkening calm. Jumping up from wherever I was sitting gave me an immediate adrenaline surge, elevating my blood pressure in seconds resulting in a return to consciousness. My body refused to give up, and I sure as hell wasn't going to go gently into the night or oblivion. Will I give in closer to my real time? When is the real time to go? Who knows?

When we die, our image always remains in the present to our children and to those we leave behind. What's more, we move on into the next stage of death as our blood congeals and our brain blanks out to return perhaps to the original vast darkness from which we originated. After we die, there's no longer a past or future for us; it's always the immediate present from which we then descend. Those left behind will always see us as we were when we died, no younger or older at that moment in our time. Our molecules go on to be dispersed and recycled just as our urine and fecal matter once did. We're all destined to rejoin that star stuff from whence we came, dust to dust. Philosophically, science and religion may have had a bad start in history, but there still may be a resolution, a joining of hands so to speak, that may give us all a satisfactory answer of the after death. That death is the final stage of a human is something religions have entertained and grappled with since recorded history.

Getting back to the dizzy spells, eventually they mysteriously decreased. The rest of my mental instabilities continued and I endured them. Whatever righted my mental listing was never specifically resolved.

Chapter 7

A Neurologist by Any Other Name

A backtrack is important at this time because of the neurologist referred to me in late February, whom I wasn't able to see until early March because of his full schedule, made an important switch for me from Lexapro to Celexa. Before the change, he explained carefully and completely what would be the difference in the two drugs. I will try to explain. Although related by chemical composition, Celexa is formulated to have approximately half the strength of Lexapro and does not have the propensity to cause constipation, in fact just the opposite, which is a condition I needed to get regulated. My digestive system and colon badly needed the break. In further reference to the change, if you were prescribed a twenty-milligram dose of Lexapro, you'd take a forty-milligram pill of Celexa for an equivalent dosage. Like Lexapro, Celexa is an SSRI, a selective serotonin reuptake inhibitor, a chemical that relieves anxiety and depression through a chemical change in the serotonin in the brain. Generally, one would see a mental change in outlook and overall better feeling within two to four weeks of taking either medication.

Though I had seen a small change in my attitude with Lexapro, but with accompanying, hellish constipation, I felt a perceptible change in my spirit, outlook, and abdominal issues after just two weeks with Celexa. The accumulative effect of having been on Lexapro for two weeks prior to Celexa and on Celexa for two weeks possibly explains why the tag-team effect gave me some final relief, plus I was expecting to soar through the depression. So in effect, I may have given Celexa more credit than it was due. Nevertheless, I was ecstatic to be on the road to recovery, however slight. I'm reporting what happened, not what I supposed happened.

After about thirty minutes in conference with this very bright and responsive neurologist, I asked him if he thought I was a candidate for a mental ward. With no hesitation, he said no and offered information about how my return to a normal state would roll out. But first, he said, "I need for you to go through a series of brain tests to remove any doubt of any sustained brain damage or a problem with your nervous system due to the numerous drugs you took, and your allergic reaction to some of them. What I'm looking for are any neurological disorders or possibly brain activity disassociation."

I told him that the only allergic reaction or trauma I sustained was with the antibiotic Tequin. All other prescribed drugs passed through me with no apparent conflict in terms of side effects. He proceeded to discuss how he needed to run several more tests in an attempt to discover any neurological disorders I may have suffered and those could be, "Nerve disorder, sleep disorder, movement disorder, and attention deficit disorder." These were nothing new, because I had had some of them all along. In other words, he needed to review the spectrum of neurological disorders in an effort to diagnose any abnormalities and treat me accordingly. This doctor had my best interest in mind.

Gaining confidence with this neurologist, I related to him what occurred with my first visit with a psychiatrist who had refused to take me as a patient. He shook his head in amazement. He felt that it was the psychiatrist's job to take on patients who were suffering with mental conditions. In other words, that's what a psychiatrist is supposed to do for a living. The neurologist was caught off guard by the psychiatrist's attitude and manner. I went on to tell the neurologist that the psychiatrist I had seen expected to have me committed. The psychiatrist's attitude and verbal discussion, mostly on his side, gave me that uneasy feeling of impending doom. In his professional mind, I was a candidate to be committed to a mental institution. Of this I had no doubt. In retrospect, he may have done me a favor by scaring me and running me off. In those frightful, sick days, my shadow would have scared the living shit out of me. That's the way it was. It may have been better to have known up front what could have been in store for me after a couple of visits with that insensitive psychiatrist. In my book, he was a real numb nut, literally.

Returning to the neurologist, he scheduled me for a brain scan wherein a tangle of wires would be attached by electrodes to my head. A brain map would be carefully digitized and resultant images of my brain would be studied at a later date. He related that the test would provide first-hand functional brain imaging that might additionally reveal quantitative answers to what had actually set me off. In other words, what made me go off the deep end.

However, because he didn't find any significant abnormalities, he scheduled yet another test, a magnetic resonance imaging (MRI) of my brain where I'd lie down, go through a short tunnel, and have a huge magnetron take photos of my brain as if it were being sliced like a Christmas spiral ham. From January 5 on, I had three MRIs, perhaps one too many. The procedure was estimated from thirty to forty-five minutes in duration. The day of the test, I developed a humongous panic attack, perhaps in expectation of the worst to come. Who in the hell knew? I couldn't fathom not going through with the test. Why was I panicking over a fairly routine test? Had I now developed claustrophobia?

The technician kept in constant contact with the neurologist who was in another building, but even after recommending two Klonopin pills, that is, a total of one milligram, I was still unable to go through with the test, much to my neurologist's disappointment, and mine too. My wife came to pick me up and took me home. She knew I'd had some issue at the imaging center when she mentioned how flushed I was and how disoriented I acted.

Horribly embarrassed by my actions or lack of mental control that day, I still went to see the neurologist a couple of more times, and he related that most of the tests he had completed on me proved I wasn't neurologically impaired or anything else. By all his tests, I appeared quite normal but still screwed up in the head, so to speak. Secretly, when I reflect on my condition, I wondered if he began to rethink my sanity. But wasn't that a vestige of my insecurities clouding my thinking?

Chapter 8

Sleep No More

Although I already mentioned my difficulty in trying to sleep at night, I found little solace in attempting to sleep during the day. I shuffled around the house during the day pretty much in a daze, wondering if this nightmare of an existence was going to ever change for the better. Death would have solved my immediate problem, but deep down inside, I didn't really want to die.

Nevertheless, clinging to any form of hope rang discordant and empty in my mind. Second-guessing my every thought or decision created an additional and enormous amount of anxiety thrust upon an already confused and anxiety-ridden soul. Calling me a self-doubting son of a weirdo would have understandingly been a compliment. And I raved on incessantly, flaunting my insanity, though privately.

Because sleep escaped me during the night, it caused me a lot of concern equally during the day. I didn't want to go out and walk, eat, or visit. I just wanted to sleep forever, and I chose the downstairs bedroom to try and catch some sleep during the day. But it was not to be. Much to my chagrin, sleep eluded me much like upstairs at night. Was there any possibility of getting any shut-eye? Several sleep medicines were prescribed, but most had side effects that further hammered me into oblivion.

Trying to find the words to describe sleeplessness failed me because that was one of the periods of minimal mental and physical activity, poor rest habits, and horrible physical side effects from the various medicines. If you viewed a roiling group of piranhas feeding on a drowned animal, then you might have an idea as to the miasma of my body and maelstrom in my mind. I reeked of fear, anxiety, and death. I wondered if I smelled then too. Was I overreacting to a mental and physical condition deeply embedded in my brain and intertwined in my body? Had I become the idiot from Dostoyevsky's novel of the same name? Absolutely not! The reality is that many of us fail when it comes to successfully or intelligently articulating that part of our sick lives. I know that bringing the truth to the surface could possibly require the skill of a hypnotist or psychologist. Bringing the turmoil to light on my own has been indeed most difficult.

For example, one day upon cursorily reading a short article on identity theft in some inconsequential magazine with respect to writing checks, my paranoid state went off like a space shuttle launched without a guidance system, especially with the recent knowledge of having misplaced my checks somewhere around the house or they were stolen. I didn't know which. This further complicated my already screwed-up existence.

With nothing but sweat and confusion, reluctantly I called my banker and asked him to close all my bank accounts but one, change all the information on my bank checks and reduce bank information to just one bank statement. With my checks, I made the change from my full name to just initials, and also dropped my home phone and local address. Using my work phone number minimized being confronted by any store or bank clerk for more information relative to my standard license ID. What I asked to be changed or deleted on my checks was completed without delay. However, for all intents and purposes, the plethora of leaflets, inserts, and information coming from the bank, if anything, increased. I worried for weeks thinking over and over how someone may have stolen my checkbook and identity. Truth be told, that really didn't happen; neither did any forged checks ever turn up. As much as I hate to admit this, later on I found the supposedly stolen checkbook intact and haphazardly stuffed in a department store bag in my bedroom closet.

One very disturbing thing that additionally kept me from sleeping in the day or night was that as I would start to doze off into unconsciousness, my heart would thump or beat irregularly for a split second, and then of course, I'd be wide awake thinking I was on the verge of a heart attack. This occurred regularly until recently, wherein the sensation seems to have tapered off.

Chapter 9

Switching Teams:
Psychologist to Psychiatrist

As this was late March and I wasn't, as you might guess, mentally progressing, yet hell-bent on getting well, my doctor again broached the subject that I needed to see a psychiatrist. I finally conceded. Not being qualified to treat me as a mental patient, he referred me to a psychiatrist who happened to be his friend. Their children played together at school and church.

Because of the psychiatrist's very busy schedule, though, he wasn't able to see me until early May. Fortunately by then, the Celexa had sufficiently reduced my depression and likewise subdued some of my high anxiety. The three phobias alluded to earlier, that is, claustrophobia, paranoia, and what I didn't know at the time was agoraphobia, came to the front as the other mental issues subsided, each waiting their turn at screwing me up and laying me on the medieval rack, so to speak. Talk about having a litany of disorders; there was no end to my medical woes.

In late April before my first appointment when Diana saw an improvement in my behavior and actions, she carefully coaxed me into taking a day trip to Asheville. I had been in the house sequestered and definitely certifiable—but for some stroke of luck missed that form of torture—for nearly four months with having taken only a few short trips to the various doctors, some with Diana while others I drove to painfully with anxiety and uncertainty. Driving for her was no easy street either, as her total left arm cast kept her on edge, but she too was ready to take a trip. Cabin fever increased our tensions, and we badly needed a break. Since early January, we had been confined to our house with only short drives to the grocery store or pharmacy. At times, it seemed like we visited the pharmacy much more than the grocery store. No mall walks or hikes for either of us; in fact, no joy or feasts reigned in our house. Our neighbors, by now catching on to some horrible next door occurrence and bad karma, brought us food, fruit, and drinks a couple of times, and we appreciated that immensely.

Diana drove us all the way up to Asheville, a small town in the mountains, and back to Charlotte the same day. Being the first trip of any consequence since early December and prior to my diverticulitis attack and Tequin, I began to regret the trip. Restless and anxious, and yet wanting to please Diana, I sat through the entire trip and meal without a fainting spell or tunneling of vision as best as I can remember. On most of the in-town trips, Diana would leave me and pick me up at some designated time. It is at this time that the possibility of getting better dawned on me. Four months had passed since the laundry list of side effects kept me at home, essentially a prisoner of my mental incapacities. I was never one to stay put for a minute and staying homebound by illness kept me thinking suicide on a daily basis. I was about to self-combust or go blind.

On the way back, Diana said, "Now was the trip so bad?" I had to admit it wasn't, but it was an uncomfortable situation for me. I really wasn't ready to enter the mainstream of life. On her behalf, I accompanied her when she needed to see her bone doctor, but I suffered terribly with panic attacks, paranoia, and anxiety that kept me on edge while my heart raced and pounded on right there in her doctor's office. Now that is really crazy not being able to stay at home, but likewise, not being able to be at a doctor's office. This was certain madness, and the dark sky and bright moon weren't even out, for the love of Pete!

My first appointment with the psychiatrist lasted close to an hour. He diagnosed me with agoraphobia straightaway, panic disorder, and other phobias I couldn't make out on my medical record copy. He recognized immediately my depression, suicidal tendency, and anxiety that was on the outs, and then asked me, "Do you have a gun in your house?" I had to admit that I did and told him it was under my bed downstairs in the main bedroom. He asked me a whole lot more questions, some relating to violence, depression, and whether I was sleeping by myself. He changed two of my prescriptions, but overall, he felt that my response to treatment and medicines would suffice to aid in my eventual recovery.

We spoke for about another fifteen minutes, and I thought he was the right choice for me. Not condescending, he did not interrupt me, nor was he given to arguments; his bedside manner was commendable. Because I seemed to draw strength and reassurance from what he related, I felt the shroud of mental illness lift ever so slightly and knew right then and there that good mental health was right around the corner for me. From that point on, we found a common ground in reading and books as a means to communicate effectively, or at least on my part. Wasn't I the one who was sick? I made a conscious effort to appear calm and not roiling in a maelstrom of confusion. I thought of a mallard swimming about calmly on a pond, while underneath its feet paddled like crazy. That described me to a tee that very day. I hoped that he didn't realize then that I was faking the calmness, but I knew that he was a psychiatrist not prone to letting a mental case fool him. I know he saw through my façade, and decided to treat me nevertheless accordingly.

His agenda to get me to a good mental health state—who is ever mentally healthy and in excellent health these days anyway—was relatively uncomplicated. Our meetings going forward became in-depth reviews of several excellent books, and one was William Buckley's book *Miles Gone By*, a literary autobiography. We spoke of Buckley's unique writing style, if not a little verbose, certainly in a poetic prose manner that separated him from many want-to-be writers. His use of the English language surpassed many philosophers and writers of our time, and he was a literary genius on a level with Germaine Greer, Bertrand Russell, and Thomas Hardy. Buckley's book drew my focus to a bead and calmed my Tasmanian devil anxiety. Reading overall seemed to reduce the occurrence of my panic disorders too, but only in combination with several correct medicines described in detail earlier in this book.

My psychiatrist kept me on Celexa, Klonopin, Lipitor, and other less invasive drugs for a little more than a year. I broached the subject the following February 2006 of cutting back slowly with most of the medicines, and he agreed as the year went on to play out. His only concern of weaning me off too early was the possibility of a rebound. That is where many of the side effects could reappear in greater force, possibly creating immunity to the very same drugs, resulting in a more difficult potential for cure down the road. Neither of us wanted to venture into that perilous and tortuous territory again, the consequences of a safe return never being a guarantee. Nevertheless in February 2006, he started a six-week decreasing dosage program that kept me from having seizures, and I reached zero dosage by early April. I had made the journey with his professional help to a drug-free state safely. Lipitor was the only drug I continued on that April, because a high cholesterol reading necessitated I stay on it.

Chapter 10

Return to Work

In late April, shortly after my ankle and thumb healed, my mind stepped right in line on a mission to heal as well. The April trip marked the line between returning to a normal mental state after enduring four months of psychosis. Keeping my mind busy had always proven effective, and so I stayed with that tactic from that moment on with knowledge that I could now focus more than say in February or March.

Speaking to my family doctor about returning to work, he grudgingly agreed, and so I returned the first week of May, still lacking that confident voice marked with authority I was noted for but otherwise fairly healthy, all things considered. I knew my charismatic voice would return in time, as I got better. Because in truth I wasn't mentally completely healed, I started on a trial basis by working only half-days for two weeks. At the end of the two-week period, I went on to full-time employment. I stayed in town, as traveling still did not agree with me yet.

Those first two weeks, although trying, allowed me to focus on things other than my phobias and illness. I derived immense satisfaction in proving to myself that I was getting better and getting back that strong voice. Working sure beat the hell out of being at home with nothing that I had wanted to do. I could read much better already, write short emails, work crossword puzzles, and not experience lightheadedness to the point of fainting. Double vision, high-volume hearing, and a lot of my anxiety were disappearing slowly. Thinking back in early April, when we went to a Queens University play, I wore earplugs, as noise and talking were so elevated still as to cause me ear pain. That was no longer true by early May.

A full night's sleep still eluded me, and my irregular heartbeats, although less perceptible, still remained, but salvation was right around the corner, I was sure of it. My cohorts and management team in as much as they sympathized with me, of course, had no earthly idea what I had endured or what had happened. As soon as had I returned to work, they wanted me to start helping them acquire new accounts, assist with the introduction of new products, or travel with them to difficult customers. It's not that I didn't want to; it's that I wasn't ready physically or mentally. The road to recovery lay in front of me, but at that moment, the road was not paved, had many holes and rocky edges, and was mysteriously circuitous.

In early May, several businesses supplying the printing industry negotiated a one-day symposium for printers who sought training for their new or inexperienced employees. Cincinnati was selected as the sight for the symposium, and the time slated was the middle of June. One of the corporate CEOs, whom I personally knew, contacted me and asked if I would make a forty-five-minute technical presentation, specifically focusing on errors in printing and how to correct them. Knowing that just a few months ago I had been incapacitated, that is, couldn't talk or walk, was afraid of flying, and suffered several phobias, especially agoraphobia, this was a quantum leap on my part, while others thought of the trip and presentation as routine. Nevertheless, I accepted. Being almost six weeks away, I saw little conflict with my condition. I'm happy to say travel to Cincinnati, the presentation, and all the meals occurred without any medical setbacks or fanfare. I did fine. I couldn't believe it. I was home free at last!

Before taking the June trip, I made three more visits to my psychiatrist and got an okay from him and my family doctor prior to the trip, and their vote of confidence resonated quite comfortably in my mind. I was humming like a practicing Hindu in a yoga trance. But was I cured now? Well, let's proceed with the story.

Chapter 11

A Smidgen of Side Effects Return

Returning to work, being productive, and working alongside my friends, while chitchatting with my relatives, immediately renewed my enthusiasm for life. Eating out became commonplace and a pleasure once more. My depression dissipating into the cosmos allowed my spirits to reach a new frontier wherein I could leave my mental illness behind. I was thrilled to be normal again, or so it seemed.

I spent the next five months never looking back and stayed busy with work, home life, and travel. Late in August of 2005, we vacationed for four days to Hilton Head and Charleston, South Carolina. While at Hilton Head, I played two hours of tennis right before noon at the Port Royal Courts. Shortly after getting back to my room, I felt faint, sweaty, and dizzy. Had my anxiety and panic disorder returned? What I was able to reconcile is that I had suffered mild heat exhaustion and came close to a heat stroke as a result of violating two important rules; I drank little water and did not rest sufficiently between sets while playing tennis in the midday sun in August of all times.

What an idiot I had been! After taking a shower, I got into bed and pretty much stayed put, not eating anything of consequence until the next morning in hopes of eliminating the dizziness and washed-out feeling. This was not so much a return to my earlier side effects as much as an unfortunate exposure to too much sun, heat, and exercise in August by the Atlantic Ocean. The southern portion of the East Coast in August is very hot and humid, definite trouble for anyone not properly hydrated or in the best of shape.

By the evening of the next day, I recuperated enough to travel on to Charleston and was grateful once again to have recovered. This was not due directly to an allergic reaction to Tequin or a total return of the horrible side effects, but Tequin had unfortunately left my adrenaline gate vulnerable to any stress. Suffice it to say, I took it really easy and, on returning to Charlotte, felt reasonably well to resume all duties.

Traveling steadily that fall and not experiencing any side effects to speak of, I reported to my psychiatrist that we might only need to meet every other week. That met with his approval.

During a meeting the following March 2007 in Memphis, Tennessee, I experienced intermittent chest pains. The pain kept me on edge and off kilter. Anxiety started in again, and I was uncomfortable. Speaking to a friend at one of the breakout sessions, whom I had known for some time and who had had a heart bypass earlier in the year, unknowingly put more fear on top of my anxiety, and I immediately called my cardiologist in Charlotte. Not able to get him that morning, I discussed my situation with his assistant, and she recommended that if the chest pains continued, I should go at once to the nearest hospital emergency room. However, in speaking to her with her calming demeanor, I felt a little better and decided my problem could be recurring anxiety and panic attacks. Nevertheless, she made an appointment for me for early the next morning, as I was to return that evening to Charlotte anyway.

Because my cardiologist was on vacation, his physician's assistant examined me, and she concluded that I might have experienced excessive stress accompanied with anxiety. She prescribed Xanax to help me with my mounting anxiety. She recommended that, although I had a stress test, an angioplasty would once and for all put to bed whether I had a blockage or not. When my cardiologist returned the following week, instead of the artery test, he scheduled me for another stress test, and it came out negative, much to my happiness. Who wants a positive test indicating clogged arteries? Much to my chagrin, however, up to that time what had caused the chest pains over those past three days was never determined, and I was left with the uncertainty of whether the continuing anxiety attacks may have been the culprit all along. The renewed anxiety gave me a glimpse of those dreaded past side effects.

Chapter 12

A Side Path of Pain
Further Complicates Things

September 2006 found me busier than usual traveling and making presentations at every turn. I was back in high demand. But now I was sidetracked with my mother, who had been sick off and on for a little more than six months. And not until she had an MRI in August 2006 of her abdomen was her diagnosis of pancreatic cancer made. The realization that she had only a few months to live hit her very hard. Likewise, it hit us all very hard, for cancer of this type was foreign in our family. In my mind, it explained what her discomfort, pain, and loss of weight were all about. But unfortunately by then, the cancer had metastasized significantly being in the fourth and final stage.

Second opinions did not vary from the original diagnosis. Surgery by this time was pretty much useless and would add much more pain and possibly a shorter life expectancy. The cancer had been diagnosed entirely too late. This is one of the cancers on which little money or research had been expended. That's changing. People such as Ruth Bader Ginsburg, the Supreme Court judge whose cancer was caught early, Apple's chief executive Steve Jobs, whose liver was replaced due to a rare cancer of the pancreas, movie actor Patrick Swayze, who died after suffering with fourth-stage cancer, worldwide known opera singer Luciano Pavarotti, who died of the same cancer, are just a few to mention whose lives were prematurely disabled or cut short by pancreatic cancer. Their illnesses have increased the awareness, and thus efforts to eradicate such a deadly cancer.

Shortly after her diagnosis, hospice was called in. At her apartment, she was put on an oxygen system and in effect prepared for the inevitable. She signed a "do not resuscitate" form, well knowing its permanent implication. Morphine was close at hand should it have been necessary. Considering she had been through a lot of past surgeries and pain with two heart bypasses and other surgeries previously mentioned, she was not at all prepared for the "Big C," as she called it. For there was always hope with her previous illnesses, but now she knew cancer would be permanent, no rehabilitation. As a spectator, yet a close son, I could see that she was highly distraught over her terminal illness. She had mentioned to me during her Christmas visit of 2005 in Charlotte that she had lost weight and felt lethargic. As I now know, the weight loss was directly related to the inability of her pancreas to release the critical enzymes that breakdown the fats and high complex carbohydrates. The many desserts she often ate that contained an abundance of sugar made her ill. Food came in and went out without the breakdown to less complex sugars her body badly needed, and nobody knew this at the time. With pancreatic cancer even in stage one, the enzymes that aid in the digestion of proteins, carbohydrates (sugars), and fats, wherein the body's cells can use them, are no longer secreted or are in very small portions, and the body eventually starves to death. This is easy to see in retrospect when one knows the signs of pancreatic cancer. Here I thought that her losing weight was normal for an elderly person of eighty-eight years of age, but I was dead wrong. Yet again, her family doctor, one trained to pick up the troubling signs of disease of any kind, had missed the diagnosis.

So in 2006, I went back and forth to San Antonio to spend time with her during her period of illness, still traveling and working when not with her. Now it was my time to reconcile her life and to put aside my meager sickness that paled in comparison to her suffering and condition, but was I prepared? Could I cope and do it?

Chapter 13

Back in the Saddle of Anxiety

The first week in November, Diana and I traveled to Arizona to attend an annual trade show at the Gainey Ranch Spa and Resort in Scottsdale. The agenda on Saturday, replete with festivities, kept us very busy. After attending morning meetings, I supervised a tennis tournament in which I also played five sets. Cocktails were served by six and followed by an awards dinner, where I gave out the money set aside for the tennis winners, myself included. Before the dance started, karaoke was opened for all who cared to sing. I sang several Elvis songs, and then we danced to great music until about 11:00 p.m. At around 12:05 a.m., in my room in the twilight of sleep, I experienced several heavy thumps in the center of my chest, all very suspiciously similar to those symptoms of early January 2005 when the whole blasted heart and anxiety issue began while in the throes of taking Tequin in pill form. One major difference, though, was that I had been off of Tequin since January 10, 2005, and here it was November 2006; there was no possible residual action this late, or was it? What was going on in my body? Immediately, I noticed my blood pressure and pulse rate increased, and I was perspiring profusely. What was not clear to me was whether I had high blood pressure and a very fast pulse before the chest thumps or vice versa. Which came first, the proverbial chicken or egg? Being in a strange place and bed, I called down to the hotel operator, and within five minutes, medical technicians were at my side, confirming a pulse of 96 and blood pressure of 186/100.

By this time, in all the commotion, Diana awoke and was shocked to see all the activity right there in our room. Nonplussed, she could not believe what the ruckus was all about, and then it dawned on her. I told her to stay put and that I would call her should I get worse during the night or whatever of it remained.

During the short five-minute ambulance trip to the main hospital in Scottsdale, the medical technician had considerable trouble finding the main vein in my left arm—and I have very large veins in my arms—yet she stabbed away in hopes of finding the right spot. Finally, she connected to my left main vein only after I advised her to thump it several times to get it to rise. Not to belabor the anxiety issue, but I had gone "postal" by the time we arrived at the hospital. I had guessed she must have been a freshman technician right out of school or something.

Admitted as a heart patient, the tests to determine if I had suffered a heart attack, not uncommon for someone of my gender and age, were immediately taken, i.e., blood work, ECG, and so on. The heart patient trauma section of the hospital was abuzz with activity reminiscent of my second stay at the hospital in early January in Charlotte, with one exception. Because Scottsdale, Arizona is the mecca of retirees outside of Miami, Florida, this hospital was staffed with doctors of every specialty known for folks getting on up there in age, especially the doctors in the heart section; they were world-known cardiologists and thoracic surgeons of incredible skills.

The cardiologist assigned to me reminded me very much of Dr. Mehmet Oz, often seen on the *Oprah Winfrey Show*, and had the same bedside manner and just as articulate; in short, exceptional. I trusted him straightaway. Surprisingly, he apologized for the numerous needle marks on my arm. Even though my blood went on to be analyzed six ways from Sunday and nothing definitively came up, he decided to give me a nuclear stress test before he would entertain the possibility of releasing me. He had not yet decided conclusively what had caused my heart irregularities, high blood pressure, and consequent high anxiety; however, I suspected he knew but still decided to be cautious. I agreed wholeheartedly. Hopefully, together we could get to the bottom of my issues.

Had I overextended myself at the annual meeting? It dawned on me that any excess exertion, whatever that meant, or stress, of what level remained uncertain, could lead to the previously manifested side effects, a return to that event horizon of insanity. That morning as the cardiologist related what would happen, he gave me the nuclear stress test, one wherein radioactive iodine, intravenously injected, traced the flow of blood through the heart to determine if a blockage existed, and he went up to the optimal settings for my age.

He said, "You're clear, but you have a mild heart irregularity probably due to an excess of adrenaline your body secretes effusively. Because of your history of allergic reaction to certain drugs, I want you to take a baby dosage, that is twenty-five milligrams of the beta-blocker Proponolol. It's a beta-adrenergic receptor blocking agent. My nurse has your prescription. Don't be too concerned or worry about its name or biochemical activity. It will help you with stress and the resultant adrenaline charge."

By lunch that day, I started taking the beta-blocker. Looking at the final hospital bill, I couldn't help but think how it looked more like a space shuttle manual than a bill. I mean, there were more entries than on a software program. A couple of hours later, I was released and back in the mainstream of life, glad to be alive. Those with whom I shared the Scottsdale trip were relieved to see me out and about and in good spirits. No kidding!

The next morning, we flew back to Charlotte, both my arms looking like pale pink pincushions, but I was back to being normal. It's amazing how much your spirits rise when you feel good and you have low stress. After taking the beta-blocker for about a week, I experienced continuous stomach aches. Reviewing the literature handout for Proponolol, one of the side effects I read was stomach upset. Conferring with my local cardiologist, he suggested I stay off of it for about a week to see if the stomachaches disappeared. They did. He then switched me to Atenolol, a slightly different beta-blocker that produced no side effects. After experiencing the positive effects of beta-blockers, it finally sunk in that they were truly the right medication for me post-Tequin. They significantly reduced the adrenaline production, minimizing the "fight or flight" syndrome so unbelievably robust in me. One of the other benefits—and not actually a problem for me—is that it lowers the blood pressure, allowing me to cope with some stress while keeping the reaction within a safe manageable range. The beta-blocker became my "magic bullet" for my active, sympathetic system always at warp speed with any fluoroquinolone. Why? Who the hells knows, but I alluded to a possible answer earlier on. The Scottsdale cardiologist broke the code for me and was in keeping with the other doctors who had correctly diagnosed and prescribed safe and low-dosage medicines until I could tolerate a higher and more efficacious dosage. Was I completely healed and able to throw away my medical crutches that were made up of anxiety, panic attacks, and depression? Only time would tell. As my system calmed down, the beta-blocker was eliminated from my slowly shrinking laundry list of medicines that I took in that time period.

Chapter 14

Dealing with a Personal Loss

Putting aside the trip to Scottsdale, Diana and I went on to Bermuda two weeks later, a trip we had scheduled six months earlier before we had known about my mother's terminal cancer. The trip, however beautiful and exhilarating, took a back seat in my mind knowing that my mother's condition teetered precariously and only blood transfusions would stabilize her condition, as she had lost so much blood to the cancerous tumor that had broken through some of the critical veins contiguous to her pancreas.

Meanwhile, I was back with a couple of side effects again: heart palpitations, light chest pains, and mild anxiety. Discussing those issues with my cardiologist, he recommended once again a week with the shoulder heart monitor. He may have been nearing his end of the rope as my internist had in my encounter with Tequin and flipping. Before the week was out, and by then November 17, I got the word that my mother was very frail, had been transferred to the Methodist Hospice hospital, was no longer allowed blood transfusions, and had only days to live. Immediately, I went to see the cardiologist where I left the monitor unit with his capable assistant. He would get back to me on the results at a later date.

Upon checking with my immediate boss and getting approval, I took a week of personal leave, ordered my airline tickets, and left the next day, a Friday, to San Antonio, Texas. Although I arrived around five in the evening, it wasn't until 7:00 p.m. when one of my nephews picked me up. I had inadvertently given him the wrong flight number;

furthermore, he had trouble locating me as the San Antonio airport was in the midst of adding another terminal, and construction had the airport personnel and traffic in virtual chaos. The confusion with gates set me back a tad, but I would cope.

My mother was waiting for me and lucid, considering she was heavily sedated with morphine. Her immense pain necessitated morphine administered under the tongue, and she needed it about every six hours. So there she was, literally on her deathbed, working a crossword puzzle and able to talk to us all. Her always-wide smile and positive attitude took a back seat under the pressure of imminent death. I took in several breaths and tried to remain calm, and we spoke for a few minutes.

I saw her in a much different light now; she was no longer the robust, endearingly animated person I'd known. She was there frail and on the cadaverously side of pale, small in her large hospital bed. Her ashen color, a consequence of having already lost considerable blood, left her mortally ill. If you can believe this, I actually feared her a little, not knowing how to act in front of her or how to articulate my below-the-surface feelings of what was happening. As quick-minded as she had always been, I knew secretly that she was in anguish and physical pain, more than anyone could relate to, and she kept her innermost feelings to herself.

She knew we were all there at her side, and she could bask if at least for a few days in the unbelievable support and attention she received from her sisters, brothers, children, friends, and extended families, for she had several, but it was momentary respite in her long life, and I had hope it would be of some consolation to her. Who really wants to die? For the first time that I could remember, back in September, she had cried and asked, "Why me? What have I done to deserve this?" I remained silent, as I had no answer.

Now in November, a few days before Thanksgiving, and by her side, I thought, *hasn't she been through enough pain and sorrow to have cancer thrown over her whole life and especially her last few days? Won't God now spare her as He had previously done for her?* I resolved in my heart that this was it, no going back, so I said nothing, and stood around like a lost soul, watching every breath she took, wondering how it was going to end for her. *Will she struggle and cry out her last breath?*

I was uncomfortable, and yet decided right there and then that I would remain calm no matter what and would be my mother's hospital advocate at her side for whatever and whenever she needed me, and I would direct all responsible nurses and doctors to carefully treat and attend to her needs. After all, she had taken her responsibilities of raising three children very seriously and never veered off the path of providing for us.

One thing that stands out in my mind while we were standing around her Saturday morning is that she wanted a picture in her room removed from her sight. "Would you move that picture from the foot of my bed and at the back of the room to the side of the room?" she said to no one in particular. What the picture displayed was a beautiful garden, but it had a large door that opened into a black void as if death were that deep, dark void of nothingness. She feared that void. Why was there such an insensitive picture there? In her imagination, festooned with religious overtones, she saw that door as a conduit to the afterlife to something entirely different. That door, she felt, should have led to a bright, dazzling entrance where Jesus Christ and God awaited her with open arms.

As the day passed into Sunday, the morphine wore off sooner between dosages, and now she needed morphine about every two to three hours. Because she remained so still, most of that day not moving but just lying in bed breathing, I felt she had drifted into semiconsciousness. Being her hospital advocate and owing her immensely, I made sure she had sufficient morphine to keep her relatively pain-free. After all, wasn't she my caretaker once upon a long time ago, when I was a sickly child, rather a parasite of sorts. In retrospect, I had supported her financially, especially in the last two decades of her life, much like my sister and brother, but had I really supported her emotionally? No. Neither did I tell her how much I loved her during her last few days when she was still lucid and before cancer made it so difficult for her to talk to us. As I looked away from her bed, in my mind's eye, I could make out the form of a brilliant red cardinal as it randomly passed over her and would hover but never light, and there I was wondering what it meant. What I did know at that moment was that I had her eulogy to write, and I whispered in her ear that I would write it and give a great one for her.

Monday morning, she awoke full of energy but somehow not totally with us, and I suspected this was the burst of energy so often seen prior to death that gives loved ones false hope that a recovery is possible. No recovery was. When I say she appeared to us to be much better, my brother interpreted her burst of energy as a sign that she might want some breakfast to eat. He offered her homemade food he cooked up earlier, but her system, unknown to him and us, had already shut down, and eating at this time was no longer a possibility.

She said to no one in particular, "I don't want any of you to trick me into not closing my casket before burial. Don't bury me alive!" In unison, we promised her we wouldn't. About ten minutes later, she went quiet again with no response, just like Sunday.

Later Monday morning, after an episode of convulsing much like a seizure, with the fire in her stomach she had told me Saturday that so pained her, I had an IV of morphine administered to her, rather than the under-the-tongue application, so that she could rest comfortably without the interruption of that Bowie-knife-in-the-side pain. She finally slept through the night, and it appeared to me she had completely slipped into unconsciousness, her chest and stomach, though rhythmically rising and falling, her last vestige of life. At 10:10 a.m. on Tuesday, the cancer silenced her body forever. Her transition to the next world was so peaceful. Back in my mind's eye, the brilliant red cardinal had gone, but it left a reminder of the bird she so loved.

Of course, I will always regret not articulating to her what I should have said early on. I'm not going to flog myself to death, because I did show my love by helping her out and traveling to see her at least four times every year. I lived 1,100 miles away, and she always showed her appreciation and thanks for the time I spent with her. It's true that she gave much more than she ever received; yet, she never made us feel like we abandoned her. I'm sure she had her moments when she was lonely, but she did have my sister who lived very close to her and helped her tremendously and much more than I could have, and my brother was there for her as well. We were all by her side at her time of final need.

I returned to Charlotte right after her burial, as it was into the beginning of the Thanksgiving holidays and flights were impossible to reschedule. I had wanted to stay on for a few more days but couldn't, and I had to keep my original flight schedule. Unfortunately, all flights were booked solid.

Chapter 15

Anxiety Déjà Vu

The New Year found me traveling no less; in fact, more as business had slowed noticeably, and it was important to secure new business if my company was going to justify several business commitments and hire new candidates to replace jobs lost through retirements.

In early November 2007, Diana and I traveled to another business trade show. Held at Saw Grass Marriott Spa and Resort, south of Jacksonville, Florida, it was close enough for us to drive there, a six-hour, comfortable trip. Suffering that week with stomach issues and taking a proton pump pill and prescribed medication, we decided to go anyway. I was sick with what seemed to me to be a mild case of a stomach virus, but I hung in there. I started to have mild chest pains by Saturday morning, as well stomach pains and mounting anxiety. *What next,* I thought?

At the tennis tournament Saturday afternoon, I coordinated it but did not play, having those sporadic chest pains and wanting to take no chances. I spoke in depth to Becky whose husband had a recent bypass and who was on the courts right then playing tennis. I said to her, "But, Becky, my stress tests and heart shoulder monitor tests were all negative. It proved my arteries were clear."

She replied, "Joe's stress tests were negative, too! But he kept having chest pains, angina like you, though with some shortness of breath, so I encouraged him to go back to his cardiologist and get an angioplasty. Are you short of breath? You may not know this, but I'm a retired nurse and have medical knowledge, however limited in the field of heart disease."

I said, "Well, I do have shortness of breath, and maybe you're right, Becky. I guess I should query my cardiologist one more time about an artery test and how I have been feeling."

Becky then replied, "Bob, to my knowledge, only an angioplasty can definitively show if you have blockage in any of your coronary arteries. In fact, Joe's angioplasty test revealed two arteries with more than 90 percent blockage in each. That same day he had his surgery. I was so relieved his doctors caught his blockages before he suffered a heart attack, even possibly a fatal one! If I were you, I'd have an angioplasty as soon as possible."

I felt much worse after the enlightening but distressing discussion, and I certainly did not let on how I felt to Diana. She'd been through enough already for Pete's sake.

That night at the awards dinner, I was a cardboard cutout of myself. I was almost too quiet, no voice again, to announce the tennis winners, but I did. To further add insult to injury, while making the announcement of the tennis awards, a tall man who appeared out of nowhere and quite inebriated walked up to me while I was speaking and took the microphone out of my hand and said, "This is the way you should make the announcement." He said a few words into the microphone. Instead of clobbering him on the head with the microphone for such a shitty intrusion, I spoke with my weak-assed tone, finished the awards presentation, slinked off to my table, ate and drank little, endured the chest pains, and returned to my room. I slept poorly throughout the night, realizing what a miserable and embarrassing evening I had experienced. The next morning, there was no improvement; in fact, I was even a little worse.

Instead of sticking around and fraternizing with all our friends at breakfast, we gathered our stuff, packed the car, and took off. Because my chest pains became much more frequent while in route, I called my cardiologist's nurse in Charlotte, North Carolina. It was a Sunday, and I knew my cardiologist would be unavailable. Describing my symptoms, she told me to check in to the next hospital's emergency room along the route to Charlotte. I told her I couldn't right then and wasn't prepared to do that traveling back to Charlotte. I said I'd call her back if I didn't improve. Well, I didn't improve. After about thirty minutes, I called her back. She was not happy with my putting off going to the emergency as she had recommended. She gave me several telephone numbers of hospitals to call that were along I-95 and I-77. Because the chest pains kept coming at random intervals, and I was struggling to catch my breath, it was critical to get to emergency immediately, as a potential heart attack was finally imminent from all physical indications. I wasn't trying to be difficult, I just loathed going yet again to the hospital for what could have been a false alarm, and I told the nurse that. It didn't faze her, and she firmly told me to go right away.

On the northern outskirts of Columbia, South Carolina, we saw the intersection for the Sisters of Mercy Hospital and went straight to the emergency section. I checked in, a nurse took my vitals, and I was assigned to an emergency room. There we waited for the emergency care doctor. He came in shortly. He looked me over, took my pulse and blood pressure, and asked me several questions.

He asked, " How often are those chest pains occurring?"

I replied, "About every five minutes."

He went on. "Are the pains continuous or do they come and go? And how long do the pains last?"

"They come and go, and they are sharp pains that last about a second to three seconds. They're like short lightning strikes."

He quickly said, "That's music to my ears. As long as those are your symptoms, you're going to be fine. You're not in the process of having a heart attack. I'd venture to say your suffering from an acute panic attack, and it is possibly why you have had a stomachache as well. That's not to say that all stomachaches are caused by anxiety or panic attacks. On the contrary, heart attacks and stomach discomfort usually go hand-in-hand. There's no need to admit you. Take it easy and go on to Charlotte. If for any reason you continue to suffer chest pains, I want you to immediately call your doctor in Charlotte and have some tests run. But right now, I'm happy to tell you that you're in no imminent danger. How's that for your Sunday?"

To say I was the happiest person on Earth and incredibly relieved would be to reveal the truth. I felt infinitely better almost immediately, but fully embarrassed that there wasn't really anything physically wrong with me, or at least with my heart. Another in the series of head issue symptoms perhaps? I was not a charlatan and had experienced a lot of discomfort and pain the entire weekend, however mental it was. We got into my car, drove onto Charlotte, relieved that the whole mess was behind us.

Even though my chest pains and the heavy pressure on my chest tapered off by the evening, I consulted with my cardiologist the next day and went in to see him as he requested. The following week, he had me take an echolike cardiogram heart test that involved a series of X-rays of the front and back of my heart along with a specific drug that induced stress without the exercise bit, and it too was negative. This was a noninvasive test and about ten times less expensive and risky than an angioplasty. I did not stress the point of having the angiogram with him. I was comfortable with the results.

All the tests both cardiologists had me take no matter if in Scottsdale or Charlotte did not show any abnormalities or heart irregularities that could produce all the aforementioned heart symptoms. Pleased with those results, nevertheless, it was still hard for me to believe in 2007 that anxiety and panic attacks could mimic an ensuing heart attack, especially considering that with those anxiety/panic attacks, my blood pressure and pulse rate increased beyond the range of hypertension, if only for the duration of the attacks. It must be considered in all the medical discussions that even momentary high blood pressure, as a result of drug reactions, anxiety, panic attacks, or other maladies, could be a precursor to a stroke. Strokes can have such devastating and permanent consequences that I don't want to even broach. I had to control my anxiety somehow. How long would these albatrosses hang on and travel with me? Perhaps it was time to get back on a beta-blocker.

Chapter 16

Death by Chocolate

After the incident in early November 2007, things pretty much calmed down from that time forward. Most of the year, I worked and traveled in the United States and Canada. I had given up travel to Mexico and South America earlier on as I kept getting a virus, cold, or diarrhea on every other trip, and so I asked to be excused from those kinds of travel locations where I had no immunity to their diseases. Late in November 2007, I flew to Cambridge, England, and on to Warsaw, Poland. I did have a mild anxiety attack in my Holiday Inn room in Cambridge, but otherwise, I felt pretty good. In Prague, just for a couple of nights, I experienced mild palpitations and anxiety, but I experienced no great degree of alarm. I took a small amount of Xanax to neutralize any side effects or episodes. I returned to Charlotte quite excited about being able to satisfactorily endure the whole trip, presentations and all.

My prescription drugs and supplements then existed of Lipitor and vitamins, no big deal. After discussing my mild anxiety experiences with my cardiologist, he put me back on Atenolol, the beta-blocker. That made the most sense. We already knew jointly from my medical history that the beta-blocker kept my adrenaline down, one of the culprits in this entire scenario.

I felt so good that in May 2008 of the following year, in my continuing corporate trips, I took a leap of confidence and flew to New Zealand and Melbourne, Australia, to assist a division of Dainippon. The Australian division needed a jump-start, and I was the person in the States chosen to train the division, and subsequently to travel to their potential customers giving product and market information. The trip took me to Adelaide, Australia, as well. Giving over fifteen hours of presentations throughout the two-week trip to some half dozen groups kept me so busy that I never really had an opportunity to think about my past medical issues, but I knew they lurked close by and would show up if I gave them half a chance. I did get plenty of rest in an attempt to keep my stress down to a tolerable degree. Without question, I paid very close attention to what I ate and ensured sufficient fiber was part of my diet. I drank my fair share of bottled water to counter any potential problems with diverticulitis. Its ugly head never reared up the entire two weeks there. Was I now sufficiently aware of what I needed to do to prevent diverticulitis and panic and anxiety attacks from occurring, or was I just plain lucky? The rest of the year went on business as usual until the early fall.

Beginning the week of September 15, I drove with Diana and Spanky, my dog, to Atlanta for a week-long, large tradeshow, where over eight thousand attendees convened. We stayed downtown and in close proximity to the World Congress Convention Center. The hotel, being one of those high rises and relatively inexpensive, all things considered, had several super restaurants. On top of that, this hotel allowed small dogs to stay, a plus for us.

It was also nice that some of my customers were staying at the same hotel. Entertaining at night was simple and pleasurable, just an elevator trip up or down to the restaurant. We took customers and their wives to Pitty Pats' Porch restaurant, next door, and the hotel restaurants for the other nights. On Wednesday during the tabletop convention—that's where you have a booth and customers come to visit and learn about new products or services—I visited several other suppliers' booths, enjoying some of their candy giveaways, and most of them were chocolates of many varieties. Being free, of course, and because my middle name is cheap, I gorged myself with chocolates.

That night I took a small group of customers to the top-floor restaurant of my hotel along with one of my colleagues, and we had a great dinner, filled with jokes, laughter, and of course, super desserts. Three of us got the double dark chocolate mousse stuffed in a chocolate icing container. It was labeled "Death by Chocolate." We ate, and that ended the evening. It was fabulous!

Around midnight, I awoke with a monstrous pounding heart, fast pulse rate, cold sweat, and felt horrible. This went on until I couldn't take it any longer. I called down to the hotel center for medical advice and was given the number for the attending medical team. I spoke with a physician's assistant, and he reviewed my condition over the phone. His advice immediately was for me to go to the nearest ER. With all the false alarms in my fairly recent past, I just couldn't bear to go through that again. But make no mistake, I was in bad condition, a bundle of raw nerves. I paced the hotel and my hotel room for what seemed like all night, although it was probably only about an hour or two. The PA and I spoke again several times; he offered me help over the phone. Not knowing my case or that I had been loony in the past, he felt confident a heart attack was imminent, and again he strongly recommended I go to an ER. So there I was, caught in the middle of yet again wondering if I was having an anxiety, panic, or heart attack. I couldn't decide by myself what was wrong with me.

I awoke Diana, who had been asleep or I hoped she had, and asked for her advice. Unfortunately, she wasn't sure either. Now I was ready to jump off the fifteenth floor and end it all.

I got back on the phone with the PA, and this time I told him all I had done and eaten that day. In explaining the whole day's events to him, it dawned on me like an elephant crushing an ant what had occurred. Although this had never happened to me in my entire sixty-six years of age, I was in the full flush and palpitations, fast pulse rate, and high blood pressure of an overdose of caffeine, a part of chocolate that can give you a false high. All that damn chocolate I had eaten, including the outstanding hot chocolate earlier that morning with extra powder as I requested, the chocolates eaten at many booths during the day, added to the Death by Chocolate dessert that night, accumulated in my blood stream. I had incurred an enormous caffeine binge. I had been tested for clogged arteries so many times before that it left me no other choice of what was wrong with me. Think of Occam's razor: "The maxim that assumptions introduced to explain a thing must not be multiplied beyond necessity" (*Random House Unabridged Dictionary*). In Carl Sagan's novel <u>Contact</u> through Dr. Ellie Arroway, she responds to a question about Occam's Razor in more simpler terms "Yes, it's the scientific principle that all things being equal, the simplest answer is usually the right one." There was no other explanation. The chocolate caffeine's accumulative effect in my blood stream was the culprit here. The adrenaline gate that Tequin had corrupted back in 2005 had not closed, nor would it ever, but was destined to remain a loose cannon for me to deal with the rest of my life. Chocolate in any quantity had never been an issue before, and I had been a chocoholic all my life with never an ill effect. Now I would need to be cognizant of how much chocolate I would consume in a day or risk the possibility of a caffeine overdose issue with all the bells and whistles of a heart attack. How much caffeine was too much was anyone's guess.

I did not discuss this with the PA. I don't think he would have believed me anyway for my age and high cholesterol certainly would lead any doctor, nurse, or medical technician to choose the heart attack rationale. I could be in for a royal screwing when the "real" heart attack would happen to me. For with it, no doubt, I would think it's just another in a series of caffeine or anxiety attacks. What a potential conflict and serious problem would be played out! I mean we all eventually die of something no matter how carefully we may take care of ourselves. The fact is the longer we live, the greater the chance is of developing one or a combination of the big four: cancer, heart disease, diabetes, or a stroke. Aging and death are preplanned and entangled in our genes. As our immune system ages, a rogue, cancerous cell coursing through our system no longer held at bay begins to multiply and replicate through our RNA, and eventually metastasizes to several organs, and the rest we already know. There's no getting around that, but I say again, who wants to die prematurely?

That morning, the PA called me on my cell phone to see how I fared. I related that I had not gone to the ER and planned to return to Charlotte that morning. In my mind's eye, I was sure caffeine was the issue. He was relieved I had not suffered a heart attack, and agreed that I should return to Charlotte and let him know how things worked out.

Chapter 17

What I Should Have Known
Then or Been Advised Of

What I know today, and should have known almost six years ago or been advised of initially by the hospital, is that Tequin and for that matter all fluoroquinolones can, depending on the patient's physical state, cause blood glucose abnormalities; that is, either lower or increase dramatically one's blood sugar resulting in two different biochemical conditions. For example, if the biochemical reaction goes to the hyperglycemic (high blood sugar) side, an excessive amount of glucose will be circulated in the blood. This condition is often benign, as long as it doesn't become chronic; however, chronic hyperglycemia can lead to organ and neurological damage. Furthermore in the process, the pancreas will secrete a vast amount of insulin to neutralize the immediate overload of sugar that is dumped into the bloodstream. But the pancreas can't do that on a continuous basis. On a short-term basis, the insulin secreted will break down the sugar so that the various organs and cells can utilize the carbohydrates. If the sugars are not broken down into simpler chains, it could cause a potentially deleterious effect on the person, as mentioned earlier.

With hypoglycemia (low blood sugar), a condition exists in which the levels of glucose in the bloodstream drop too low to fuel the body's activity. Symptoms here resulted in my constantly feeling weak, being hot and sweaty on occasion, confusion, dizziness, and on top of this, having a very rapid heartbeat and blurry vision. All of these manifestations were mentioned in more detail in earlier chapters.

One of the very disturbing things about fluoroquinolones in general, i.e., "Cipro or Tequin is that they increase insulin release from the pancreatic islet cells. As a class, therefore caution maybe warranted with all quinolone antibiotics. Based on post-marketing data, disturbances in blood glucose may be more common with Tequin (gatifloxacin) than with other fluoroquinolones," according to the *University Health Care Hospitals and Clinics* (February 17, 2006).

From a Canadian study involving Tequin (gatifloxacin), "The use of Tequin has been associated in the rise of blood sugar abnormalities (Dysglycemia). These abnormalities are not restricted to patients with diabetes. Studies indicated a 4 times increased risk of Hypoglycemia (low blood sugar levels) and a 17 times greater risk of developing Hyperglycemia (high blood sugar). These abnormalities are brought about by the drug interfering with the regulation of insulin secretion from the pancreas. Other side effects include kidney failure, heart attack, stroke and seizure." This is according to an article from the March 2006 N*ew England Journal of Medicine*. Unfortunately, no hospital ever shared with me that I had low or high blood sugars even when I asked for liver and blood tests results. I had no way of knowing if their failure to mention the results was neglect, a mistake, intentional concealment, or a conclusion that I was not capable of understanding the results.

Unbeknownst to me at the time Tequin was prescribed, "Public Citizen, the public interest group founded by Ralph Nader, filed a petition with the Food and Drug Administration demanding a Tequin recall. The petition made reference to 388 patients with blood-sugar irregularities associated with Tequin, including 20 deaths and 159 hospitalizations since January 2000" (FDA Alert Side Effects, June 19, 2006—Tequin(gatifloxacin).

Did my Tequin side effects have roots in biology and psychology? Because my condition was never treated as a cause-and-effect by the hospital or any of the doctors, especially with my second and third hospitalizations, it was clear that I was on my own and had to come to my own conclusions. Considering I was two cards short of a full deck, or at a minimum perceived as such, the possibility that they would join me in a concerted effort to tag Tequin as the culprit was about as remote as life existing in hot volcanic magma. So the truth is that it could have been both. I've learned that everyone has something considered poor health or poor health habits. You just have to learn to accept and cope. We all eventually die, but good sustained health will allow us to live a longer and fuller life.

I can think about it all now and almost laugh at my physical and mental conditions that, for the most part, were concentrated in about five months, and after that time many of the unfortunate side effects eventually disappeared the following year. Anxiety, sequestered in my brain, can unpredictably creep in today if I try to do too much in terms of something physical or if I watch a stressful, fast-paced action movie or TV program. I know this to be true. It's as if the adrenaline gate between my adrenal glands and my sympathetic system never completely closed but has remained crack-happy open. The gate opens wider if I allow stress to burden me, and gobs of adrenaline flow out. Consequently, I am on notice now and careful not to allow that sort of thing to rear its ugly head, or I pay for the unfortunate outcome and have trouble even catching my breath. As a crutch, I keep a few anti-anxiety pills handy in case of such an episode; in fact, they're too old now and probably have lost some of their potency. Since May 2005, I've not had a recurrent panic attack but have experienced several bouts of anxiety, which I discussed in length in several of the previous chapters.

Did I age over that year? Of course, and I now have permanent wrinkles in my forehead and face that can be easily ascribed to the pain and numerous anxiety and panic attacks endured. The vast amount of drugs I had to take just to get back to before when I was eating gumbo-okra soup that 2004 New Year's Eve have added to my aging. My hair has fallen out some but can be ascribed to Lipitor as one of its minor side effects, but who really knows? Okra soup, most nuts, and chewy things I avoid like the plague, or for sure I masticate them until there's nothing but puree left to swallow. There's no use tempting those pockets lining my colon where, when particles of food get trapped in them, harmful bacteria begin their uncontrolled, unwanted growth and result in pain, disease, and fever.

Before I leave this chapter, I want to refer back to an IV titer in Chapter 2. Therein I mentioned that a slow titer of a medication through an IV allows the body to accept and thus tolerate generally whatever dosage is administered. I now know that had I equally been given a titration schedule with Tequin in pill form; that is, wherein one starts with a low dosage and then it is gradually increased, this whole mental aberration episode may have been prevented.

After leaving the hospital with the initial diverticulitis attack, I was given an immediate one-thousand-milligram pill twice a day. It's as if I had never had the first dosage of Tequin, or more like the antibiotic had accumulated in my system to such a great degree as to cause damage to my system.

Chapter 18

Walking a Tightrope or One Mouse Click Away

How my mental condition played out is a situation for another book; nevertheless, it went like this: Think of a dog that on a whole as a family dog is well behaved, eats, sleeps, and plays with its master. On occasions, the dog will get completely out of character and will act, quite unexpectedly, like a wild dog that is unbridled. He will take a toy, a favorite master's pillow, or some valuable object and tear it apart or break it to pieces. He never means to do it, but the feral dog gets into him, and he has little control but to let that enormous energy vent out. I was like that feral part of a family dog for the entire five months. I was a raw, open wound of unbridled energy, in disarray, unfocused, and destructive, yet not violent. Had that state lasted any longer, I would have been committed to a mental institution. I discussed my mental instability with my doctors and some relatives, wherein I desperately tried to reveal little in the process—like they didn't know I was "loony toons"—and asked a lot of questions. There's no doubt that I was one mouse click away from being committed. However, it's important to relate that you must have an excellent family doctor who networks successfully in the community of skilled doctors and uses them for his referrals. On my behalf, his role and influence were very critical in my gradual ascent to sanity. I may have not thanked him adequately for his successful role in ensuring that I had the right doctors to rehabilitate me. He was understanding and patient with me as his patient.

It's difficult to keep reminding myself daily, if not sometimes hourly, that to keep diverticulitis at bay, I must drink a minimum of eight glasses of water each day. That alone keeps me minimally purged, and I eat many vegetables and mainly chicken, turkey, or fish, and they go through me quickly. It's all about getting what you have eaten through your digestive system every eight to twelve hours or less. A small dosage of a beta-blocker keeps my adrenaline flow to a minimum, and thus heart rate constant, while tempering my anxiety and minimizing a chance of palpitations. My blood pressure has stabilized to around 120/60 and pulse rate steady at around 60, not bad for an old fart. Yogurt, the low-fat and low-sugar type, at just four times a week stabilizes my abdominal flora, and garlic with some of my meals on other days puts to bay any bad bacteria multiplying indiscriminately that could result in infections. Which one or ones work effectively, I can't tell you, but garlic has been considered the Russian antibiotic for centuries and appears to help me when I get a flare-up, as indicated by pain in my left side.

So that's how it all started that New Years' Eve day. How do I live today? I live on a very thin tightrope. I fear diverticulitis will return with a vengeance one of these days, and it won't go away no matter what antibiotic derivative I take. Again, my antidote today is a conscious effort to drink an abundance of water every day and consume a lot of fiber, perhaps eighteen to twenty-five grams per day. On occasions, I'll eat as much as a bale-of-hay a day to get sufficient fiber, just kidding. But seriously, I do eat around 30 percent or about eight grams of fiber for breakfast. That way I'm better prepared to deal with the rest of the day with less stress on fiber intake. The other absolutely helpful thing that I do to regulate my system is to walk and/or hike from twelve to twenty miles every week during all seasons.

One other consideration is that I often wonder if the severe constipation that I endured for almost a month while in that five-month duration may have contributed to a relapse in hernias on both sides. Each hernia had been repaired many years earlier and went on to be repaired again in 2009. My right indirect inguinal hernia reappeared sometime around 2004 to 2005. A more specific date eludes me. Furthermore, I have had four hernia operations in my lifetime, three more than most men. Other than that I seem to be okay, wink, wink, nudge, nudge; get that bird off my shoulder will you?

Chapter 19

Final Outcome

After twenty deaths and over 179 hospitalizations, of which two hospitalizations were mine, not counting the first emergency trip due to the January diverticulitis bout, Tequin was removed from the pharmaceutical market in May 2006. Although I spoke to several professionals and others about the Tequin debacle and whether I should sue, I decided to not file a claim with the manufacturer of Tequin. At my age, I'd probably not live to collect any damages anyway. What's more, the energy, time, and expense to file the claim through a reputable legal firm would not be worth it considering most legal firms end up with the bulk of the dollar award as related in many cases. That may not sound fair, but the media has portrayed the legal system as the ubiquitous winner in many medical cases, and I believe that. Why else would the legal profession pursue such a claim if not for a large settlement? The published word seems to hold the benefit of the doubt for the masses, and we believe what the media says is gospel, however inaccurate they may portray the events. Who checks on all the specific data or sources for accuracy? "Not me!" said the blind man.

One conclusion that stands out in my mind, however medically accurate, is as follows: If a drug precipitates a mental illness, another drug or drugs in combination may restore and stabilize the out-of-balance chemistry, as was in my case. But if a person becomes mentally ill through a gene issue, i.e., heredity, or by a family misfortune, like the death of a close relative, it's much more difficult to treat and finally cure, and the illness may take more time, effort, and drugs to correct.

Furthermore, the disabilities of many young people, whether mental or physical, directly caused by Tequin live on unfortunately. In my case, which I mentioned before, I still suffer some anxiety, and once in a while palpitations. I continue to have tunneling vision on occasions, and I do have trouble periodically with my right foot. Maybe this book should have been titled *My Right Foot*. I do practice relapse prevention and alluded to that sequence of events earlier on. Caffeine, in any food or drink, I singularly reduce to minimize any palpitations or anxiety, and that is unfortunate, as I love chocolate almost as much as my dog. As you can imagine, I loathed visiting the Tequin disability site on the Internet for fear that the condition could mysteriously reappear out of nowhere, or that I might just get another anxiety attack. I certainly don't want to jinx my issue; "knock on wood," as they say.

So you ask, does Tequin still haunt me? Yes, I did not come away unscathed. Nevertheless, there's nothing like the passage of time to erode ill feelings or a memory of ill health, in my case both. It seems now like a vague dream that occasionally struggles to surface in my mind. So what did this whole episode cost me in terms of money, forgetting personal time lost, which was a lot? It was in excess of ten thousand dollars and includes, but not limited to, ambulances, medicines, and copayments more than I can possibly count. More important was the total cost for the insurance companies, and I would estimate that to be in excess of sixty thousand dollars.

Further to my consideration of the final outcome, did any good come from this aberrant adverse reaction? Yes! One of the aspects of this whole affair is that I have not suffered a migraine, vascular, or tension headache since December 2004. Removing most sugar and caffeine from my diet around January 10, 2005, clearly began a period of purging my body of those needless things, along with harmful environmental toxins that invade our food, soil, and the air we all breathe. Drinking sweet tea, eating pastries often, and drinking sodas almost every day prior to December 2004 contributed to most of my discomfort, such as headaches, bloating, and weight gain. In 2004, I weighed right at 168 pounds. I now range from 159 to 162 pounds, summer and winter, respectively.

May the unfortunate abdominal illness that hyper jumped a physical condition to a real psychosis precipitated by an antibiotic stay sequestered forever. It was hell, an unfortunate nightmare, and a veritable drug-induced descent into an event horizon from which I did fortunately escape, but only through the help of several highly skilled and conscientious doctors.

About the Author

The author has written over twelve short stories, fifteen technical papers published in several magazines, over 50 poems, and is the winner of NAPIM's Pioneer Award in 2001 and the TAPPI Bettencourt Technical Award in 2007.

Cantu worked for thirty-eight years in the chemical industry. Now retired, he lives part of the year in Charlotte, North Carolina, and the remainder of the year in Blowing Rock, North Carolina, where he writes, hikes, and stays active as both an amateur astronomer and naturalist.

About the Book

What appears to have been a miracle antibiotic drug to relieve the painful symptoms of diverticulitis proves to be problematic as an adequate treatment. Cantu goes on to experience many debilitating side effects from the drug. The antidote is worse than the original condition. The result is mental illness that plagues him for two years while under medical treatment. Only through the combined skill of several doctors does Cantu escape the black hole of permanent mental illness.

www.ingramcontent.com/pod-product-compliance
Lightning Source LLC
Chambersburg PA
CBHW022103170526
45157CB00004B/1463